I0448499

Rhythms of Reality

Solving the Mystery of Life with Yoga Meditation

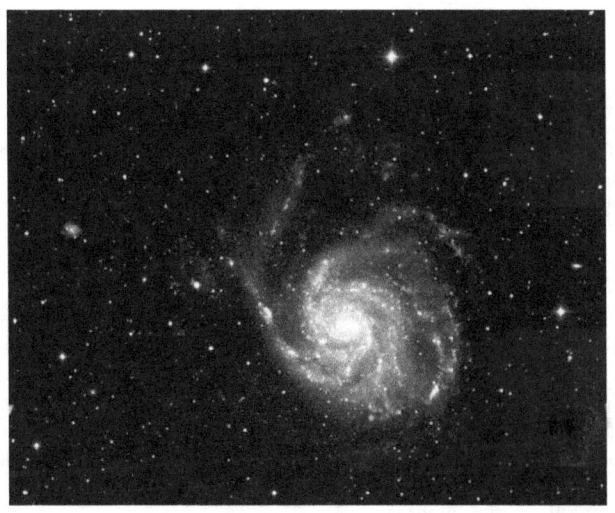

Stephen L. Ryan

Rhythms of Reality

BookSurge™ Publishing
First Edition Printing: 2005
Second Edition Printing: 2011

ISBN-10 # 1-4196-1927-6
ISBN-13 # 978-1419619274

Printed in the United States of America

* * *

This book is dedicated to my amazing wife Daniele and incredible son Skylar.

* * *

This is also dedicated to you, the reader.

May you realize the source of life, and create a life in truth.

Let that truth become your eternal reality.

* * *

Rhythms of Reality

CONTENTS:

Introduction

You were born and raised in a certain place with specific circumstances. Probably, you became educated on how to interact with others, and also get a job. Inevitably, you also learned some things which you have no use for, maybe even habits that work against you. Perhaps you became enamored with entertainment, technology, news, sports, finance, religion, relationships and politics. You may have become busy with family, career, and recreation. Nothing is wrong with this process, and it's not your fault even if there was. However, there may have been a time when you wondered if there was more to life. You may have realized there are things going on that you do not understand. Certain events may have occurred which upset you, or that you thought wasn't fair. Maybe you just have some questions. Isn't it odd that the first things we should be taught when we come into this world, we are not? How strange it is that we arrive and no one informs us where we're from, how we came here, or why we are here. Eventually, as we develop we begin to realize that there are pieces missing in our story. Some people realize this but then due to a lack in energy abandon questioning, preferring to stay at their current level of conscious awareness. When we do realize and ask others, we often find most people don't know, or will act or speak like they do; but then it becomes clear that they are only perpetuating myths that

1

they themselves either don't understand, or only think that they do. Many people are simply unable to believe it is possible to find the answers. You and I are different in this regard. That is why you are reading this now. You intend to increase an understanding of the mystery and purpose of life. When you buy a new car, it comes with an owner's manual. If only the human life came with one as well. Here is an opportunity for us to create one together. You have been brought to this book because in some way you have questions and are seeking answers. This may be a conscious or unconscious seeking. This book will attempt to answer those questions. It will do so in a non-denominational manner which does not impose a specific doctrine or moral judgment. Instead we will examine the nature of "Reality" or "Truth," (which are the root of all questions), in a logical manner, thus generating deeper questions within you. You will be guided to the answers to those questions and find that there are actually no questions without answers, that in fact you are the primary question itself and the primary answer. This statement implies that an aspect of you is Reality, and thus the answer to the question of reality is also in you. This seeming dichotomy is possible based on the inference that who you perceive yourself to be at this moment is only a portion of the whole of your being, which is actually the real and complete "you." The primary question you seek to answer is three parts:

1. **Who am I?**
2. **Why am I here?**
3. **What is the purpose of life?**

The primary answer to who you are will reveal a greater understanding of Reality. You will be challenged to expand or confirm your sense of self and your perception of the world, thus exposing the source of eternal happiness and success in life. Specific techniques will be outlined which will provide you with practical tools you can utilize to make your "true self" the best it can be. By doing this, you will have done your part to make the world a better place too because you are an integral part of this world, and the entire universe.

Caution: There are those who try to impede our efforts to find the truth regarding the nature of Reality. They are the ones who have not asked the same questions yet. Thus, they want to disable our ability to have the answers as well, lest we find them and have power over them. This is a fear-based paradigm. Fortunately, fear-based motivations never lead to lasting success.

If we are to begin questioning Reality, we must start by questioning its origin. Whether or not you believe there is an absolute Truth, there is certainly enough evidence to justify examining the subject seriously, rather than just disregarding it out of laziness or disbelief in the possibility in finding an answer. Not doing so implies one cannot be bothered to look at the evidence. If there is enough to make it worth examining, to claim that there is not, sounds like one has already made up their mind without doing the research. We would be wise to investigate for ourselves and make up our own minds about it. Some have said, "Don't listen to those whom claim to know the Truth, because there isn't one." At first glance, this statement that we cannot know, and that there is not one universal truth, sounds very humble and tolerant. However, if you ponder the intention of this statement, it is a contradiction.

To state that there is no such thing as Truth, is itself a claim to be the truth.

So, is it true for everyone then? In that case, it is proclaiming itself a universal truth as well; the very thing it denies exists. Or, is it only true for the person stating it, but not for us? In that case, it doesn't make any sense because it would be a relative truth and not an absolute one. To say that we do not know the truth is an assumption that the person stating it knows everything because it rules out even the possibility that we could know. How can a person know enough to be sure that others cannot know anything? Although at first glance it sounds very tolerant, like a "wolf in sheep's clothing," it is remarkably intolerant towards anyone who disagrees with this statement. They are essentially saying that everyone has a right to their own beliefs, except that we do not actually have a right to believe our beliefs or to think that they are actually true. The result is that those whom do believe in Truth in our present society are mocked, or at the very least, not taken seriously.

This entire world, real or not, is certainly something and something cannot come from nothing.

In my research over one hundred metaphysical texts have been examined. I have done my best to extract the fundamental core wisdom from what I considered the most significant of them. The information has been condensed, reorganized, interpreted, and presented with a contemporary and systematic approach. This is a new simplified interpretation of an ancient and complex philosophy. The information contained herein is timeless and entirely relevant. It is hoped that this book can serve as a comprehensive, yet concise and practical reference tool for those consciously and actively on the journey to increase understanding of the true nature of Reality; or at the very least seeking a way to experience peace, love, joy, success and an end to suffering.

It has been said that Truth does not need to be proven because those who are ready, will intuitively know it when they come across it. If not, then they were not ready. Yet, I feel that there may be those of us out there who are ready enough on a different level. Some people may be able to accept certain concepts, but only if explained in a logical progression, thus leading them toward deeper realizations through reasoning and via a secure foundation intellectually, rather than by faith alone. Although I may agree with much of the many texts I have encountered, I believe that unless a person is guided in this way, they may eventually switch paths repeatedly, thus becoming increasingly confused and further from the truth they seek. They may even abandon their search altogether due to a lack in progress or understanding. That is why this book raises certain questions, then uses reason to introduce ideas without them being forced upon anyone. This way, one can be exposed to concepts without feeling that they are being imposed as mandatory doctrines. This should allow one to feel comfortable to explore the information without feeling obligated to accept it. I believe that in this way faith can develop but will become less likely to be shaken later.

In this book the words, "Truth" and "Reality" are used interchangeably. We all have variations of what we think is "real" based on what our minds perceive in the world, and that perspective is what we each consider our reality; but if that was the only definition of reality, then each person would be experiencing their own, rather than sharing one with others. Events may seem chaotic, coincidental, or even at times inconsequential, but closer examination reveals a universal order in how life develops, progresses, and declines in a virtually incomprehensible, interdependent manner. Ultimately there must be one universal perspective for all of us which we've been unaware of. It is that reality we refer to as, Truth. This is what is meant when people state that they are seeking the truth regarding life. Finding this Truth answers the previous three questions: "Who am I? Why am I here? What is the purpose of life?"

In order to answer these questions, we first must believe it is possible to. Next, we investigate the matter of truth regarding Reality. Consequently, we will proceed to examine the evidence of reality, its origin, and its relationship to you.

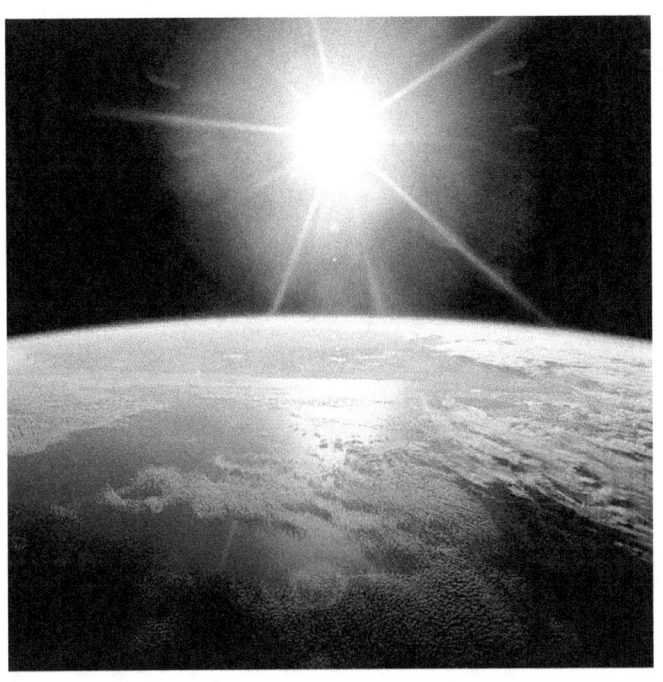

Chapter 1

If you observed the world around you closely, perhaps you have noticed there seems to be some unseen force which binds it all together. There appears to be some invisible cohesion causing things to appear as they do. Is it Time? In part, but time is only the factor that allows us to experience events in a linear sequence. Time is essentially a component of perception. Is it Perception then? Not exactly, if it were, then life would seem far more chaotic then it already is. It would be more disjointed, like a dream or nightmare. Since our lives seem to include others experiencing the same events (reality) as us, it must be something else. (We will revisit the concept of dreams later.) The evidence we seek is all around us. We simply have not examined it properly. We must look at the images in this environment more closely. All matter as we see it appears solid. Mountains, trees, and chairs, even your physical body all appear separate from each other; yet matter actually consists of nothing solid at all. Science has proved this, although most people haven't realized the significance of it yet. This world and everything in it is nothing but empty space with atoms buzzing busily within, constantly changing. The rate of motion collectively produces a certain vibratory frequency. Furthermore, the difference between these objects is simply a matter of slight variation and combination of chemical elements. Most people only believe what they see, but our eyes are only tuned to a certain common frequency (rate of vibration). Ergo, our vision is extremely limited, and so is our perception of reality. The dictionary definition of reality is essentially stated as: "That which is unchanging." So by this definition, the world as we presently perceive it is not entirely real. That is why the mystics of the East refer to this world as being an illusion. An infinite network of atomic rhythm is the underlying structure of our so-called reality.

It's all about energy.

Energy is vibration, or activity. Any kind of activity must be preceded by thought. An apple cannot be eaten unless one first has a rapid succession of thought: Hunger for food, thought of the apple, then of how to obtain one, and finally the act of consuming it. Thus, it is clear that all energy begins with thought. When you look at raw nature, the Earth, plant life, insects, animals, weather, volcanoes, plate tectonics, the ocean, evolution and all the complex functions carried out within all of these subjects, (not to mention the incredible ballet of planets, solar systems, and infinite galaxies all moving about each other in mathematical precision); and all of these harmonic actions being executed without our conscious control, we must wonder: "Where is the force of thought, the source of intelligence, that we know must exist, originate from that could orchestrate this incredibly diverse rhythm of life?"

Everything seems to exist solidly. This is due to our sense perception; without the five senses, could not be perceived. The energies are attracted to each other thereby producing the illusion of form. The sense of sight and the consciousness that interprets what is seen allows this perception. These days, we would be foolish to deny the fact that there lies nothing else on our skin except hair, for with the aid of powerful lenses, (which can be thought of as seeing different frequencies than our eyes are able to), we know that our skin is in fact covered with billions of helpful bacteria. With more refined vision and intellect we would realize that everything is not the way it appears, but actually pure energy moving through each other with no real divisions at all. Energy we begin to see is vibration. The highest vibration is light. Science has demonstrated that faster than the speed of sound, is the speed of light. The mind is an incredibly complex and advanced machine that scientists estimate we still only use about ten percent of. This mind did not become created accidentally and all the thoughts you have, and the sense of who you think you are has come from this mind. Since this brain was not created by chance, using this logic we can infer that there is intelligence beyond our mind, which is the creator of it. This "Creator" I refer to can be labeled with whatever name you feel comfortable with. For the purposes of this book we will interchangeably refer to it as, "Spirit," "Soul," "Life,"

"Truth," or even "God." The source of thought we now see is not the mind but Spirit. The process of creation as we know it being: Spirit/Consciousness > thought > light > vibration (of varying frequency) > elements, minerals, atoms, and molecules, which compose all that we know presently, and can even be traced back and grouped into five common properties: Ether, air or gas, fire, water, and earth.

There is actually much more going on than we have been aware of. Everything around us is actually a complex living energy in constant motion. Certain objects such as rocks or plants seem to be inert or lifeless because their speed of growth is at a different rate. If we were to record these objects over a long period of time and then watch the video at a faster speed, we would see plants grow right before our eyes. We would also observe that apparently inert rocks form crystals, which actually grow too. Plants also evolve and adapt to their environment just as so-called higher forms of life such as insects, animals, or even humans. Certain plants, when not able to get the nutrients they need from the soil due to changes in the environment, adapt by becoming carnivorous such as the Venus Fly Trap, which developed a way to catch insects (in its mouth) and digest them. This shows how everything is conscious life and energy. Through examining the evidence around us, we have further realized the impossibility of this universe and ourselves in it occurring by chance. Subsequently, we have acknowledged the existence of a higher power at work because this energy is clearly being guided by a creative intelligence which we have still not fully understood. We now recognize all that exists is composed of variations of chemical elements which are all energy in motion, and essentially one force perceived at various frequencies. Since everything is composed of this primal energy, naturally so are we. Have you ever examined yourself, including your mind? Obviously, all of our bodies consist of the same basic properties, yet somehow no two individuals look exactly alike, not even twins. So even though we are made out of the same elements, we seem to have individuality, but we know that we are more than our bodies, after all we have a mind. We believe this makes us even more unique. Most of us believe this is who we really are. However, do you realize that there is probably not one thought that we can think that has not been thought of before by someone else at some point in time? To be more specific, look at our likes and dislikes. Look at our beliefs, at our taste in appearance and lifestyle; do the media and collective consciousness not program them all into us? What brands do you like? Why do you like them? Is it because they were the highest quality and best price? Or, is it because of the advertising? Is it because everyone else has the same thing? What is considered attractive? Is it not what we see in the media? The fact is, if you study the subject you will be surprised to see that there are virtually no thoughts you have about any subject that are actually your own. I can assure you that whatever topic we discuss, if we study our responses we can trace the source of our knowledge which we have presumed to be our own opinions, to have come from elsewhere. Perhaps something someone told us or something we read, and where did they get it?

We are all recycling the same thoughts through each generation. The only difference between us as people are slight differences in physical appearance and a different collection of thoughts which we have accumulated based on what we have been exposed to in life. If you rewind your life so to speak, and everyone else's, and started over giving everyone the exact same life situations and experiences, and exposed them to all the same stimuli (programming), how different would we appear then? This train of thought is meant to force the question of who we are by making us realize we are not who we thought we were.

At this point it may seem that I am trying to make you seem less than what you believe yourself to be, but this is not the case. Most people are not happy all of the time. This suggests that we want things to be a certain way but have not achieved that. Or we have achieved what we thought would make us happy only to find that it didn't. Therefore we are confused on how to produce the results we believe will make us happy, or we are confused on what it is that actually does make us happy. This confusion about life and how it operates further suggests that we must also be confused about ourselves, and our relationship to life in this world. Therefore whatever we thought we knew about ourselves, and the world, must either be missing something or be completely incorrect. Hence, in order to shift our perspective to an accurate view, we must first unravel the false notions we have held on to thus far. We do this by examining our properties deeper until we reach the source, as we have done just now. At this point, however, we have only gone so far as to unraveling the physical and mental aspects of being. It would seem that even being given all the same circumstances and experiences there may still be something that makes us different. That something must come from beyond what we have looked at so far. Even if we entertain the notion of a person having numerous lifetimes, we still must arrive at the same question of the source of the original life. This is why you can see I am not intending to make you feel inferior. I am attempting to show that whomever we really are, while is much more conditioned and limited physically and mentally than what we have thought previously, is actually much more than either of these. We see now that to find out who we are, we must look further, we must go deeper. Finding it, we can empower ourselves to make our own choices, and live with true freedom.

Most people think they are the body and mind only. Such persons who think they know themselves have only found their ego. Not ego in the case of being inflated as the so-called ego maniac, but the self in the deluded state of thinking it is nothing more than the sum of the parts, a false idea that it is a separate entity from everyone and everything else. Due to this misconception we spend our time imprisoned in dualities of temporary happiness from fulfillment of desire, or suffering from loss or inability to obtain the object of desire. We do this because we erroneously believe that we need certain things in order to be happy. Since we are under a spell of separateness we look everywhere endlessly for it, everywhere except within ourselves. You are able to smell a flower because you have a nose and the sense of smell within you. We derive some happiness from objects only because we have the happiness already within us also. We are searching indirectly for it. There must be a more direct approach.

We spend all our lives seeking happiness outside of ourselves and this is why we can never stay satisfied, becoming bored eventually with everything. One gets to the point where the senses are over-stimulated seeking pleasure and this always leads to frustration, disappointment, and unhappiness. This is because everything in the world constantly changes; objects of desire are impermanent, as are we (the ego). We are born, and then sleep half of our lives away, we work at jobs we dislike most of the time, we suffer, get sick, and then we die. Most of our time is spent at work. When not working, one spends time only struggling between the states of getting angry at desires unfulfilled or fulfilled but then lost. One also spends considerable time in fear of losing what is possessed whether that is the objects, goals, status or body. All this caused by ignorance of the true nature of self.

Everyone is unsatisfied with their lives in one way or another. Most are only pretending to be successful or happy. Everyone suffers from a mass delusion that there is a level of "heaven on earth" to be achieved. They will struggle a whole lifetime trying to obtain it, but consider: Do you really think that if you searched the whole entire world over, that you could find just one person who was rich, healthy, happy at work, (or on permanent vacation), sexually satisfied in every way, completely uninhibited, attractive, never bored for one moment, possessed everything they ever wanted, and never lost anyone they loved or cared about? Only this person could be free and happy. Well, even if this person did exist, how long could they maintain it? After some time they would certainly get old, probably sick, and definitely die. Certainly along the way this would also happen to those whom they cared about and that's not perfect happiness. It is an impractical dream. There is nothing wrong with having a dream, but perhaps we should try to use our will to achieve more wholesome goals. We try so hard to achieve a temporary physical perfection for ourselves that will not be reached, and if reached, not maintained. Yet, if we put half the time and energy into methods of recovery, we could become immensely rewarded. There must be a feeling much greater than any that can be gained by any material means and is everlasting. Do we not really seek a state of pure bliss, ever-new joy; one with knowledge, peace, love, success and infinite consciousness? We must have the ability to escape the painful cycle of death and rebirth, transcend the mind and its limitations and become truly liberated beings eternally; true wealth and peace at last.

Our true self cannot be the temporary personality, which we identify with now because the definition of reality is, "that which is unchanging." Since you are constantly changing, then you also, are not real. If you and I are not real, then what is real? If who we think we are is not real, how is the non-reality supposed to be able to recognize the actual reality? Since this is a world of duality, if we label something as ugly, it can only be because we have an opposite to that label such as, pretty. Therefore, if we are discussing the subject of non-reality then we can deduce by this association that there must be an opposite of non-reality, which would be, reality. If we were stating that this outer world is changing and by definition, ultimately unreal, including our bodies and minds, then we can see that looking to the inner world would be the logical place to search for reality and our true selves. We have stated that the outer world, which is unreal, is a world of activity, cells in constant motion. Hence, the logical method to look within to the inner world would be to maintain a state of inactivity. If we are able to discover methods to maintain a state of inactivity, what then should we look for first in attempting to find this reality we speak of? Perhaps we should look to the substance, which everyone naturally seeks. Since everything here that we know in its natural state is beautiful and ingeniously designed, what force could permeate all of it? Why does nature work so harmoniously, and what force holds it all together? Looking at our world we observe the laws of nature such as gravity, magnetism, planetary orbits, and physical attraction. One quality can be seen to be the common root energy of these. Could that quality or substance be *love*? We all seek it in one form or another. Even a criminal may love what he/she does, although society does not approve. What "force" causes animals to care for their young? Based on this reasoning, it becomes clear that we are all seeking love, but through outward means. However, this outer world as we know is temporary, and so the love we search for is fleeting and will never truly satisfy. We seek love from people, from things, from activities and everywhere in the outside world. Is it not evident that the answer to who we are is within us, beyond the false self? Can we not assume this true self may actually be the source of love, joy and wisdom? There must be a happiness which is permanent, pure, never boring, better than any achieved through the material world, and therefore absolutely real due to being a constant variable. I propose the possibility that this is who and what you really are. I propose that by looking within, you will go beyond the false self which is based on the exterior; that by going within and re-associating your consciousness with love instead, you will be able to differentiate between what is real, and what is not. What looking within means is that the world around us, which we see with our eyes and also perceive with our other senses, seems to be outside of the physical body; However, going within does not mean that we are to somehow look inside our organs and skeleton for the truth we seek; What it means is that as we have already understood thus far, the world we perceive consists of energy in constant motion. This energy moves at various frequencies. These frequencies are classified as different levels such as atoms, molecules, infrared, and ultraviolet radiation. But science neglects for the most part to include the unseen in this classification. We cannot see the wind, but we have other means to prove to ourselves that it exists. Also, we can't see emotions, yet does anyone doubt that they exist? These emotions are also energy. They can even be classified and incorporated in a scientific-like scale of energy. For example, it seems logical to surmise that sadness and anger are negative, and therefore a very low level of energy. Accordingly, love would appear to be at the top of the scale as a very positive energy. If we know the world outside of us is all energy from levels we can see, to levels which we can't; we can safely assume that some of these levels, such as those of emotions, are actually in us as well. When you hear the term "go within," this signifies inverting your attention from the distractions of the outer world, and focusing that attention to the energy of your own body, inside of it. So we are not talking about the physical inside, but the energy inside. Since all energy is a vibration, it is quite simple to become aware of this inside yourself. Certain techniques to accomplish this will be introduced later. How does this energy awareness enable us able to locate the core of love we hypothesized earlier? Because since love is also energy, by concentrating on a base level (of our energy), we become increasingly aware of higher, more subtle levels as our perception develops and becomes increasingly refined until eventually reaching the most elevated state which may be experienced as love.

In order to prove or disprove this concept, you must accept it as you would if given a new pair of glasses. You cannot know if the lenses are clear and if they will improve your vision unless you try them on. So try this perspective on and let us continue to reason and perhaps we can unravel the mystery of existence and see Reality more clearly. If we are love, and if that is the nature of the Soul, then we were also obviously created with love. We were given the ultimate gift as well, which is freedom. The freedom we have is to appreciate our existence and experiences, to give our love, or not. What kind of life would we have if we tried out this perspective and found it to be true? What would a life be like to be in a state of total contentment and love without fear? Can we believe in the possibility of a life without fear? Is it possible that what really limits us, is simply ourselves? Isn't it time to upgrade our belief system, since the beliefs we have held to now have not worked for us as expected?

Some people have the belief that there is a judgmental, demanding and punishing Creator. But is it not preferable to believe in a loving one who is not like us in that respect? (Assuming we wish to think of God as a separate entity.) But let's say for a moment that God was judgmental and life is a test. Would it be fair that some people come into the world with monetary wealth and other favorable circumstances, while others come in poor and abused, but at the end of the finish line, both are equally judged? That doesn't seem fair or even make sense. What about the fact that babies already have personalities and traits different from each other before they could have a chance to be developed by reactions to life experiences? Why are some young children so talented, and others not? Wouldn't a more logical assumption be that these qualities are not distributed unfairly by a judgmental cosmic dictator, but rather they are acquired through experience and practice in former lives (reincarnation) and the effects of previous causes?

Attributing positive and negative factors in life to a God unfortunately inhibits us from assuming any responsibility for our lives. Even if there are certain unavoidable events or opportunities, which are assigned to our particular life-time, certainly we also have the ability to choose. We always have the choice of how we will react to these circumstances. Since we already know events are played out due to the cause and effect of our actions, we can see that our reactions to certain stimuli will result in certain effects in the future. That being said, we are essentially creating the future. If we observe nature, we will see that life is a cycle. The seasons change but do not end, the sun and moon revolve in orbit but do not end. Where one life seems to end, closer examination reveals a connection as the declining life yields and contributes to the new one. Need I elaborate on infested corpses or fertilization of the earth by bodily decomposition? Human life is also a cycle. Although usually people do not remember their dreams, we couldn't say that people do not dream. Correspondingly, even though some people may not remember their past lives, that doesn't mean they have not had any either. As for those who think there is no life after death, I will only point out that as mentioned, everything in life suggests a cycle and there is no evidence to suggest that at the highest chain of our evolution, it would simply end. The idea that all this brilliant creation, functioning to geometrical rhythms which we don't even fully comprehend, could have no meaning is absurd. It is obviously an ingenious design to say the least. We know that we have not created all of this (including ourselves), but something must have set this all into motion. This vast, infinite intelligence that is responsible for all that we know (and do not yet know) simply must have a reason. Therefore we will not even justify this concept with further elaboration; especially because one of the key goals of this book is to answer the monumental question of the meaning, purpose and significance of life. Based on the assumption that there *is* meaning, we will proceed.

Unfortunately, those who are not yet aware and are thus still sleepwalking through life, to them it can sometimes seem more like a nightmare instead of a dream. They attribute the events of life to being lucky or unlucky. To them there can be no control over the creation and they take no responsibility for themselves. Not to say that we have 100% control all of the time. I don't think we do, at least not at our present state of evolution. The reason for this is that we are not alone. Our desires must be coordinated in linear time with others. But that having been said, does not mean we cannot have increased control and success and/or happiness. Globally speaking, the weather seems beyond our control. But what if I suggested the possibility of the weather being greatly affected by the collective, chaotic thoughts created by the population of our world? What if we could balance ourselves and harmonize society to a peaceful coexistence? Perhaps the weather would become tame and mild. What if we each achieved the ability to concentrate deeply, and unified our will power? What could be accomplished? Instead however, most humans experiment (possibly through many incarnations) of pleasing themselves using the senses to fulfill desires and suffer numerous pains and disappointments in life. This process repeats until we remember the truth of our origin, our purpose for existence and its relativity to the whole. At that point we realize the need to change our view and seek the means to do so. If we find the means, we can practice them until we have proven the validity of these ideas. By "means," I refer to actual methods to balance and harmonize our being with nature. This includes techniques of going within to perceive the higher levels of our energy and consciousness. The validity in doing so is proven by the state of well-being, contentment, peace, love, joy, wisdom and success that we can assume would be the result of practicing diligently the proposed methods.

When you look at all the world's qualities in its pure form, before being corrupted by humanities' unbalanced, inharmonious use of reason and will power, everything is truly beautiful and created with true wisdom. All great works of art are created by their master's love for the process. This love is what inspires the artist's power of deep concentration necessary to achieve the greatness required for the immense details they depict. Thus, we can also assume that we were created with the same love. True love is expressed as freedom, and we have the freedom to love or to not love. This further shows us that whatever intelligence created us and the world, loves us the most and that all is held together the way it is by way of love, due to our freedom in choice of expressing this quality. When we act selfishly instead of with love for each other, we go against universal laws of nature and suffer consequently not because we are being punished by an angry god, but because we are acting against our own best interests.

It seems that a person suffers until they realize on some level that there are effects caused by actions, which we generate. These effects are either positive or negative corresponding to our actions. We develop an inclination to avoid the negative and an affinity for the positive. Only after much experience do we see that there are probably no coincidences and that seemingly disassociated circumstances are all inter-related and specifically assigned to us based on our "Karma." That is to say, we are the cause and we experience the effects of our actions. Where others see coincidence, I see consequence. As we said, it is not the result of a judgmental deity, bestowing blessings on favored ones and punishments on others. It is simply a matter of us experiencing the consequences of our actions. These are the results of all our actions, and it may take a long time before the proper circumstances come to fruition in order for us to finally experience the effect. This creates the illusion of coincidence, or things happening beyond our control. The illusion is linear time. Then, we actually attribute this to a greater being. If we are creating our own outcomes as explained regarding karma, then we are in this regard, our own god. Since essentially we are (a part of) God, why would we judge or punish ourselves? We are experiencing things, which we planned to, so why would we judge ourselves based on our own expected reactions? If Spirit is all knowing and powerful, how can it become angered as though something could happen against its will? We are the creators of our experiences and the experiencers of our creations. Thus, "we are the makers of the music, and we are the dreamers of the dream." We are sleeping gods within our own dream. As a result, we realize that if we want to experience only positive effects, we must generate only positive causes. In seeking the methods to remove suffering, people have often looked to some kind of institution such as a church.

There are many religions in the world. Some may have been formed at one time by enlightened individuals who expressed to others the truth as they perceived it, and how to reach it by using their own techniques based on their own personal experience of what worked for them. Different people therefore choose certain religions based upon certain similar traits. But what is "true" religion? A true religion should be able to teach a person how to commune directly with Spirit. They should not just interpret scripture or preach about it. Today it seems that most of the heads of the various religions are not truth realized "gurus;" this is why the meaning and purpose has been forgotten and many people have become averse to religion. Some are participating out of mere blind belief, social pressure, or even habit. Some religions are even based on wrong views such as prejudice or may manipulate their devotees for their own motives, as with cults. A true religion must bring the follower to experience the truths for him/herself and have a direct understanding of Spirit. It is not necessary to join a particular religion, group, or guru. Yet, you may feel inclined to do so, as there are some benefits in surrounding yourself with like-minded people. Your environment is an important factor in development. Although one may transcend their surroundings, it is beneficial to have people with similar aspirations nearby. Many cults exist in our civilization led by egos, which can notoriously twist the words of Truth to suit their own purpose. That is not to say that there are no genuine teachers in this world, but none of them are perfect, and one should not follow blindly. Beware also of anyone that makes you feel that you need them. Since you came in to this world (and will leave this world) alone, you do not "need" anyone.

When a person has been led to the proper methods and becomes adept at cultivating self-balance and harmony, in time they become in tune enough to allow more direct communication with Spirit, the higher intelligence which created your mind. This communication is what we have referred to as, intuition. These are moments when the universal true you, (Spirit or Consciousness), communicates and you understand intuitively. In other words, the perfect-self speaks truth, peace, love or wisdom to the imperfect-self, just as you would soothe and comfort yourself (or a loved one) when injured. It's almost like the advanced you of the future came back in time to help the confused you of the present. When something is intuited to occur, and it does, do we glimpse the future and become aware of an event about to occur? Or, did we create the happening and then observe it, as it became a reality? This is a Divine Dichotomy. Since there are many levels to our being and all time is ultimately relative, could the answer be that both are true? One part of us creates and another part perceives/experiences. Think of what we call Spirit as: the source of all being, the source of peace, love, joy, wisdom, success and truth. All things are created by this and therefore, all things are rooted in it. That is everything, and everything is love. By being love, you become everything. Ergo, by being everything, you need nothing and are free to be; thus, literally a human being. When we finally become dissatisfied with anything this world has to offer and we realize there lies much more behind this illusion, we are guided to that which will aid us in finding our way beyond it. You may have received guidance to the methods of being still and looking within through a series of events, circumstances, books, intuition, or people that you meet; (Maybe even guided without an external stimulus.)

Although we are in the habit of attempting to acquire temporary joy from the impermanent, it is knowledge of eternal joy that we really seek, perhaps unwittingly. However, if instead you look within for what you seek, you may find that joy is who you are, the core of your very nature, the substance of your Soul, its very essence. If we stop seeking permanent joy from impermanent persons, objects and activities of the material world, we would find what we seek in the stillness inside ourselves. I can say this is true for me, as have many others, but you must discover if it is for you. Once realizing this as true for you, you realize you need nothing outside of yourself to be happy. Remembering yourself as the very source of all you have been blindly seeking, communication now has a new purpose: To communicate joy through simply being joy. By being in joy, you will enjoy everything. Others, who still seek outside of themselves for this, will see themselves reflected in you, and recognize themselves as the very same. The circle is complete. We are one. Could this be the truth you are seeking? To be free and "Self-Realized," that which obstructs our awareness of the true self must be removed. The truth must destroy the ignorance. Forgetting who and what you really are, (the All in all), creates the illusion of needing something outside of yourself to be happy. This creates desire and fear which both trigger anger. The inner knowledge of living the untruth leads to guilt, which leads to self-judgment. This in turn leads to a subconscious expectation of being punished, which further feeds the cycle of ignorance, desire, fear, and anger. The cure for all of this as stated is revealed by the knowledge that we are one, and the One is itself, joy and love. To reiterate, it is this perspective, which is referred to as Truth.

Ignorance of our true nature causes desire, fear, anger and sadness. These also lead to several main afflictions (sufferings) including: guilt, imbalance, uncontrolled thoughts, and uncontrolled emotions. These afflictions make us feel powerless because we become slaves to them, which further contribute to a separation mentality. Here is a clear way to identify the problem and focus on the solution.

The *Cause* of Suffering "Equation"

**IGNORANCE > DESIRE > FEAR + ANGER (and/or)
SADNESS = Guilt + Imbalance + Suffering.**

- **IGNORANCE** = IGNOR-ING THE TRUTH OF SELF BEING THE SOURCE OF LOVE AND WISDOM, ERRONEOUS BELIEF OF SEPARATION FROM THAT. (LEADS TO DESIRE).

- **DESIRE** = SEEKING JOY OUTSIDE OF THE SELF IN THE IMPERMANENT WORLD, HAVING ATTACHMENT TO OR EXPECTATION OF PARTICULAR RESULTS. LEADS TO FEAR & ANGER. (CAUSED BY IGNORANCE).

- **FEAR** = AFRAID TO NOT ACQUIRE OR OF LOSING THE ACQUIRED IMPERMANENT JOY. THE OPPOSITE OF LOVE. (CAUSED BY IGNORANCE AND DESIRE).

- **ANGER** = AGGRESSION DUE TO RESISTING THE LOSS OF THE ACQUIRED, OR IMPATIENCE WITH OBSTACLE(S) TO ACQUIRE THE DESIRED. (CAUSED BY IGNORANCE, DESIRE & FEAR).

- **SADNESS** = DEPRESSION DUE TO RESISTING THE LOSS OF THE ACQUIRED, OR FEELING POWERLESS OR VICTIMIZED TO ACQUIRE THE DESIRED. (CAUSED BY IGNORANCE, DESIRE & FEAR).

- **(Guilt)** = SHAME AND/OR REMORSE, A NEGATIVE, OPPRESSIVE FEELING. (CAUSED BY SUBCONSCIOUS KNOWLEDGE OF LIVING AN UNTRUTH AND RE-ENFORCING THE IGNORANCE OF A SEPARATION MENTALITY INCLUDING: DESIRE, FEAR & ANGER.

The *Cure* of Suffering "Equation"

**TRUTH > DISCIPLINE + DETACHMENT
(With Aware Action) + DEVOTION (Love) +
FORGIVENESS + CONCENTRATION >
MEDITATION = Balance + Peace + Joy + Wisdom >
Freedom/Self-Realization.**

You must know some key terms in order to understand why humanity suffers and how it can be remedied. Awareness of truth inspires us to attempt to remain cognizant at all times, in all situations. We can practice discipline, detachment, devotion, forgiveness, aware action, concentration, and meditation to bring about peace, joy, wisdom, and eventually full self-realization. Let's review these terms and definitions.

"The Truth" is that you/we are part of one eternal consciousness. The One is pure and infinite Joy, Love, Peace, & Wisdom. You are the source of everything you seek and the creator of your life. Does this feel true for you? If not, perhaps it will become so. If it has or will become true for you, does that not mean it is true for all? Are we not all essentially the same? What could happen if we accepted this as truth? Wouldn't we essentially be immortal and no longer fear death? Wouldn't we then be free, truly able to love life fully? What could happen if we do not accept this as truth? Wouldn't everything remain more or less the same? Have we been happy to seek endlessly for happiness, only to become disappointed, time and time again? Aren't you reading

this because you are seeking an end to suffering? This philosophy can work for you because it has worked for many others. Try it and see. Will it be an easy fix? No. It works because it takes work to practice the philosophy and the methods. With the right attitude it will not feel like work, only effort. Everything in life requires effort. It requires effort just to get up in the morning. Is it worth it? Only you can decide. Why should you bother? Because you have been down this path before and you know where it leads. Isn't it time to try something else? The difference here is that this path may be better and this path being better, may never end. Being aware of yourself as the source of all you have been seeking sets you free. "Need nothing, enjoy everything;" this is the antidote to ignorance.

Discipline is living life in harmony with nature. We must discriminate what affects us positively or negatively and refrain from the negative, cultivating the positive. We must find and follow methods which will counteract the ignorance of a separation consciousness. Because we have been living in ignorance of cosmic law for so long, we have developed inharmonious habits, which cause our imbalance and suffering. To change our way of thinking and life-style habits seems difficult, and the ego resists. That is why changing to realign us with nature and lead balanced, peaceful lives requires effort and is referred to as a discipline. Eventually this will feel natural and become seemingly effortless. This discipline also includes practicing methods such as those being outlined now and those to be introduced later, which lead one to living a balanced life with full awareness. This is the antidote to imbalance.

Detachment is using discriminative wisdom to break the habit of expecting and desiring joy from sources other than you, by realizing the truth of the inner joy. It is quite all right to have things, but not to believe you own them. Things come and go but they are not the source of your happiness. Joy is permanent and constant, infinite, eternal and ever new. Not expecting or needing particular results counteracts desire, fear and anger. This is because the only moment that matters is this one right now. We can act with intent to accomplish things but if we want to do this without suffering, we must act also with detachment. This means we should use all our faculties and abilities for achievements, but accept whatever results occur, knowing that a higher intelligence has determined what is, or is not, meant to be at that time. If we were more in tune with this higher intelligence, I suppose most or all of what we attempt to accomplish will come to be, since the ego will not have misguided us in the first place and we would intuitively know what should, or should not, be done in a given moment. For example, perhaps not everyone can be a rock star at the same time; who would harvest the crops, or clean the streets, or teach in school? That is why practicing detachment helps to align us with Spirit, because we learn to let go of the little self and its selfish desires. We re-associate our consciousness with Spirit and act on behalf of the greater whole. In this moment, things will be whatever they are. Desiring them to be other than what they are presently will cause suffering in the form of frustration or anger. Since now can be the only real moment, desiring things to be other than they are in that moment is to be resisting reality. People say: the truth hurts, but it is the resisting of truth that really hurts. Only by accepting things as they are, do we enter reality; and only by entering it can we empower ourselves to change circumstance. We become empowered when we are fully present in the moment. By simply being, we are being present; by being present we experience our presence. Experiencing this presence is to feel our unity with all that is. Being all that is, is being able to manifest what currently isn't. What we resist persists because if we don't acknowledge something exists, we cannot change it. How can you change something that you believe does not exist? Only after we admit something is there, are we able to do anything about it. By detaching, we learn to, "let go and let God." Trusting that a higher intelligence is maintaining order in the seeming chaos brings peace. This aware action is remembering these things, or at least trying to at all times. Even though you may be detached from the desires of the world, you can still enjoy participating in it through desireless action and bringing joy to others by being the source of joy yourself, and not expecting anything in return. The wonders of planetary nature provide sustenance for our species without expecting anything in return and there is peaceful harmonic balance. Correspondingly, we should also give without expectation of a return on our investments. This allows us to shift our consciousness to enjoying the process itself rather than the result. Awareness of our true nature and acting from this state of being allows us to avoid ignorance. Practicing methods to cultivate peace in oneself through detachment may just mean learning the skill of doing the best you possibly can at all times, without having any expectation whatsoever of anyone else having any inclination to do the best that they possibly can at any time. Detachment is the antidote to desire.

Devotion is love of and allegiance to the truth of unity and inner joy, and commitment to living the truth. This counteracts the guilt that results from a mind which fears the wrath of an imaginary punishing god, or the wrath of nature as a reaction to the subconscious knowledge of transgression from harmony. Everything we think, say and do should be done with love for ourselves, for others, and for the process of life, which is Spirit itself. This is the antidote to anger and fear.

Forgiveness of the past and of any person, thing or circumstance you feel that has caused you pain in the past is an aid because we realize that being ignorant of knowing the joy within is the only real source of pain. We all have been subjected to the disease of ignorance at some point. Now that we realize this, we can use compassion to try to maintain an awareness of the eternal source of joy by avoiding ignorance. We are then able to forgive ourselves because we remember separation was created in order for us to experience the reconnection and appreciate our truth more profoundly. Being aware that the joy in you is also in everything else makes you a part of the whole. This enables you to forgive others also, because the others are also you. That is why we can say, "We are one." Being love means to love yourself, as well as others, since you and they are one. To be free from the guilt of separation, you must bring all life together and reconnect with the power of forgiveness. By forgiving yourself for the ignorance of the past, and also forgiving others for their transgressions, you release everyone from the cycle of judgment, pain, and retaliation of negativity. Nothing is really personal. All negative actions are simply creatures acting out, based on ignorance of our nature. You would not want to drive a knife into your hand because you know it is yours, and it would hurt. When you realize that you and another come from the same source and are actually one, you would not want to hurt another either. Of course that doesn't mean that you shouldn't defend yourself or others (if needed) against an ignorant and dangerous individual. It's the intention that matters. But you must also be careful not to use this to justify negative actions deceiving yourself that you have good intentions. You will no longer be angry with persons or situations because you no longer take things personally. You are not even simply a person, you are Spirit, and Spirit is the first cause of all life, and since you are one with this, you also must be the first cause of forgiveness. This means that you must not wait for good to happen to you before you are good. This means that you must be the good you would like to see in the world without expecting others to do the same, or even to start it. You must be responsible for taking the first step in forgiving others. Express love in order to experience it; others will become affected energetically by your positivism and eventually reflect that. If everyone were to be responsible for themselves and discipline their thoughts, words, and deeds to exude only good energy, then the entire world would instantly be peaceful. Perhaps the reason bad things happen even to good people is because this is the result of previous bad actions both individually and globally. It is all systematic, non-personal fulfillments of cause and effect. These could be things done in this or a previous lifetime. What we should be learning from this may be that when we do good things, we feel good. When we do good things for others instead of ourselves we feel good because the others are ourselves also. What goes around literally comes around when the proper circumstances come to fruition. It is wise to cultivate goodness because happiness is what we are all after. So, the question is, how do we feel good? The answer is, to do, say and even just think good things. Be the first cause of goodness, and you will feel good. As a result, others will then feel good, and the world will respond with goodness for you. Then after quite sometime of this, when all your negative karmic "debt" has been paid off, you will be truly free. This is the antidote to guilt.

Concentration is to focus on something with complete attention and eventually with practice, to have no distraction. When this concentration is used to focus on the inner joy of being, this becomes meditation, which constitutes a part of the methods alluded to. This breaks the cycle and instead re-enforces a return to Truth, assuring avoidance of returning to ignorance. This aspect will be elaborated upon soon, when we explore the methods of discipline. You can see that by controlling the mind, we become empowered to choose what we think and feel rather than be a victim to an uncontrolled mind and world. Therefore, this is the antidote to uncontrolled thoughts and emotions.

Please refer to the below chart as a summary and practical reference tool.

THE FREEDOM FORMULA		
The Cause >>>	**>>> The Cure >>>**	**>>> The Result**
Ignorance of truth >	> Knowledge of truth >	> Truth is realized
DESIRE >	> DETACH & DEVOTION >	> PEACE
	(With aware & loving action)	
FEAR >	> FORGIVE & ACCEPT >	> LOVE
ANGER >	> FORGIVE & ACCEPT >	> JOY
SADNESS >	> FORGIVE & ACCEPT >	> JOY
IMBALANCE >	> DISCIPLINE >	> BALANCE
Guilt & Suffering >	> YOGA MEDITATION >	> SELF-REALIZATION
Physical imbalance >	*> Proper exercise & diet >*	*> Health & physical control*
Emotional imbalance >	*> Proper breathing >*	*> Emotional control*
Mental imbalance >	*> Positive thought >*	*> Mental control*
Disharmony in life >	*> Positive & aware action >*	*> Harmony & happiness*

The methods of yoga and meditation and their ultimate culmination with Self-Realization are to be introduced in an upcoming chapter. Although you will find that the science of yoga incorporates these traits above, it is a very complex, detailed and involved process. The above formula was created in order to simplify the problems of life and depict a clear and direct solution with its result.

Our fall into delusion and ignorance is a complex issue and so is its reversal. However, the root of all problems in life stem from desire, therefore the most important remedy is practicing detachment. You may choose to learn about and practice yoga, but find many obstacles along the way. While the goal of yoga is to balance, purify, and reconnect us consciously to our true self ultimately, you will encounter difficult situations that test your ability to practice. You may wish there were something more specific to stop the pain immediately. The good news is that there is something. We have discussed the need for detachment, now we will reveal how to practice it. But be warned, it's so easy, that you may disregard it, thinking it's too easy to be true. That's your ego talking. Just ignore it, try it and see. The more you do it, the more effective it becomes and the faster it works. One day, as the effects of yoga reach fruition, you won't even need it anymore.

We have stated that the root of our problems is desire caused by ignorance. This refers to a lack of knowledge regarding the true nature of the self. This lack of knowledge means there is no awareness of reality. From this we can infer that the method of detachment will be a technique designed to bring about awareness. Since we have been erroneously focused on the outer conditions, this will be an awareness of the inner state. The first step would be to focus on the body, the outer shell so to speak, of our being. Not being body-conscious per se, such as concern with appearance, but a deeper awareness. All material things including the body are manifestations of energy. Furthermore, energy is manifested and manipulated by thought as we have already seen. Subsequently, the next step of awareness is to focus on the energy of the body. The way we can do that is to become aware of the breath. By focusing on the breath we can disassociate from the body and go within. Doing so, we can realize the source of breath, which is also energy. Therefore, by focusing on the breath we become aware of the energy. This new awareness frees us from the limiting body and ego identification and allows us to connect with an expanded sense of self. We soon experience that sense of self as peace, love and joy. Finding this, it becomes irrelevant what is occurring in the outer world. Yoga takes this simple technique we are about to mention, much further so we will not elaborate on it now. The reason we are discussing this here is so you don't have to wait to finish this book in order to start experiencing an end to suffering. You see, it's all fine and good to talk about the Truth and discuss the practice of an art and science to perfecting ourselves, or even speculating philosophically how we already are Spirit, and just need to remember this, but that doesn't help us right now. The next time you are stuck in traffic and start getting angry, or if your loved one leaves you and the pain is overwhelming, philosophy isn't going to help a lot. We need a practical technique. We need something to ease the pain immediately.

We are assaulted by unpleasant or painful emotions, thoughts, and sensations almost constantly. So many in fact, that we just accept it. Most people don't even believe there is something they can do about it. Some people believe there may be something and research it as with this book, (like you). Some people receive the methods and don't believe, or believe but don't use it. Will that be you? Well, if you are tired of suffering, I guess not. All these problems are really in the mind. The body sends a signal to the mind, which then has an idea about it and reacts with emotion. But so far this inner cause and effect has been without our direct, conscious control. We have been slaves to our mind; however, our mind is just a tool. Since we know that the mind alone is not who we are, how can we get past it and then control it? First we need to detach from the body, right? We need to become aware of the energy under the body and mind, right? So how can we do that? Just like the body and mind, the breath is also energy in a more subtle form. If we pay attention to the breath, we forget about the body and mind. As we practice watching the breath, we experience it becoming calmer and calmer until we almost feel that we do not need to breathe at all. Then we start feeling a deep peace. This stillness between breaths is the peace. Breathing then almost becomes a nuisance. Then we start to notice the vibration which permeates the body. The mind simultaneously becomes calm with the breath because they are connected. This still calmness becomes your center. In this stillness emotions subside, and the pain dissolves. As you then gradually move your awareness from the breath to the energy, you begin to feel the sense of yourself expanding. That is because the same vibration in you is in everything. By becoming one with vibration, you become aware of your oneness with everything. With practice, you can begin to realize the possibility of controlling this inner energy, but that aspect will be discussed in greater detail later in this book as part of the upcoming yoga chapters. For now we can use this technique to experience instant peace in a situation that causes us to suffer in some way, however great or small. Imagine being able to choose the thoughts and emotions you have anytime, in a given moment rather than be a victim of circumstance.

MEDITATION TECHNIQUE: Detachment

1. Sit straight if possible so the energy can flow freely within you. Remain still.

2. Close your eyes and exhale completely, pulling in your abdomen to squeeze out all the air as though you were ringing out a sponge.

3. Inhale slowly through the nose (the mouth is closed), deeply filling your lungs. Do not strain yourself.

4. As you inhale, count mentally until you reach the limit of lung capacity.

5. Begin to exhale slowly also through the nose, and also counting mentally to the same number. Pull in the abdomen once again to expel all the air.

6. Be sure to have the count of inhalation and exhalation to be the same.

[Example: Inhale to a count of 12 and exhale to a count of 12, for 12 rounds if possible.]

7. Release control of the breath and breathe naturally. Do not control it. Continue to sit straight with the eyes closed and remain without motion.

8. Simply observe the breath flowing in and out of the body. Watch it in a detached way, as though you were observing someone else breathing.

9. Do not worry about time; forget about it, there is no time. There is nothing you need to do and nowhere that you have to go. Let go of the body and just be the "watcher."

10. As the breath moves in, think the word "Om," which is a verbal representation of energy. Being the root sound of all words, it comes closest to recreating the sound of this energy. This also helps to detach from the thoughts and the mind.

11. As the breath moves out, again repeat, "Om," The deeper significance of this word will be explained in greater detail shortly.

[Do this for at least 10 to 15 minutes after the 12 times of controlled breathing.]

Doing this simple form of meditation creates a balanced rhythm and forces awareness of the present moment. Physiologically, it makes you feel pure and light. Psychologically, it makes you feel peaceful and in control. Spiritually, it is the beginning of awakening to the truth of eternal bliss. Immediately, it is a tool to deal with pain. This technique is only the basis or beginning of meditation, but for now, it is more like your medication. If you have never done this, you may be surprised how effective this easy technique is. It may be a first indication of "proof" for these ideas of Truth. This is how we can begin to practice detachment, which leads to deeper meditation. Although this may be a quick fix for day-to-day dilemmas, we still need to practice other methods if we want to become balanced, end the pain and experience Spirit permanently. That will be outlined later. For now, we will return to the topic of Reality as we continue to attempt to uncover the reason for our being here, the how and why of it all.

Is our experience here governed by Destiny? Our lives are pre-ordained only by what we decided to experience while we were a part of our greater (higher) selves prior to physical birth. It should soon become apparent that our lives may include situations allowing for us to experience the general ideas we had before we arrived on this world, but we are still free to make new choices, create new opportunities, and thus change our "destiny." Therefore, we will now study further the nature of our existence and consider the reason(s) for it.

Chapter 2

As explained earlier, the world consists of people, animals, plants, and objects made of atoms and molecules all moving endlessly, constantly changing. Every cell in your body is completely different than the ones you were born with; even your tastes, opinions, attitudes and style have changed. Which means that if it is all changing, what is real? When you dream, that seems very real. In fact, the only reason you know it isn't is because you are not able to share your experiences with others. But when you wake up here, and experience an event, you are able to talk about it with others and confirm that it actually happened. (Although, I suppose in a dream you can dream that you are having these validations also.) I guess another way to prove this world is real would be that things seem to happen as a chronological sequence of events. If you remember, your dreams while at the time seeming real, in retrospect they are disjointed, illogical, and out of order. So we are always moving back and forth between two dream-like worlds, one seeming more real than the other. So, why do we need to sleep? The answer must be to recharge, right? Yet, even though a car needs fuel to drive, it doesn't need to "sleep." Since we eat food for our fuel, why do we need to sleep? The act of eating alone does not supply us with enough energy to maintain our physical existence. Technically, the process of food digestion actually uses energy before it releases it. We also derive energy from breathing, and even from the sun; yet even these are not enough. If eating, breathing and sleeping were the sole sources of energy to maintain life, then we would be able to give these to the dead and bring them back to life. Obviously, this wouldn't work. Deducing from this, we can see there is another source of life which science is still too undeveloped to explain. We can observe that we are passing through three states of existence: this wake state, the dream state, and the unconscious sleep state. We already know what happens in the first state, you reading this right now, for example. We have also already discussed the dream state. Although during sleep, much time is spent dreaming, why is that the majority of our sleep state is not remembered, as though we were unconscious? The third state is the secret we need to unravel. No one talks about it; it is taken for granted as a part of our nightly routine, yet it remains a mystery. As you may already know, or are starting to realize, you and I are not of this world. We are literally from out of this world. Our Souls entered here at conception and developed a fleshly covering and a filter of thought which we call our mind. We developed egos, which are our acquired personalities. We developed these in order to adjust and cope with the illusion of separation from our true existence and self. We were born with five organs of sense which function in conjunction with the mind-filter to perceive the objects of this realm. We continued to grow, adapt and learn. We have experiences and memories, desires and fears. Eventually the momentum begins to decline and physical old age develops. We eventually become sick and then die. Perhaps at this point our Soul returns to the Source, reflecting on its experiences in the body and in the world. The Soul then may reside in other worlds or dimensions where it incurs the good or bad consequences it accumulated through its actions in the world, before finally returning to a world like this again for continued experience. At some point the true self, who is the Soul or Spirit, could start emerging through all the false layers. Questions arise such as, "What is the meaning or purpose of life?" This questioning awakens a process where events start to lead one in the direction of discovering reason and functions of Life. During one of the lifetimes which you experience, you may come across literature such as this book, which may assist you in revealing this and discovering methods you can use to facilitate or even expedite the realization of Truth. One method originating from India is known as, "Yoga." But before we get into that, let us wrap up the mystery of sleep. During the mysterious third state of deep unconscious sleep, your Soul is returning to its Source temporarily; the true and natural state of being. While in the world, that experience is your only true state of peace, and re-energization. Without going there, you cannot continue to exist in this world. That's the way I see it. So why don't we remember returning to our source? The answer to this is actually also the answer to the greater question regarding the meaning of life. Why do we incarnate here, forgetting our true nature of immortality and consequently suffer through life with only fleeting happiness?

Since the truth is in everyone, isn't it accessible to all? Isn't it odd that most people do not know the truth of their own being? Isn't it ironic that someone would be mocked for being audacious enough to claim to actually know who they really are, and why they are here? Consider that your true self could actually be the co-creator of the universe. Like a totem pole, your present state of awareness is at the bottom of that pole. At the top is your highest state of awareness, which you currently feel so disconnected from that you give it another name, as though it were separate from you and more powerful than you. But our experience of who we think we are at this time is confined to our limited perspective. We are like the fingers on our hands, and each of these fingers thinking that they are completely separate entities from the other fingers and even from the hands themselves. If it were true, that we have a separation mentality, why would it be so? The logical conclusion appears to be that we are ultimately one unified consciousness. This Spirit seems to have separated itself into individual entities, which have descended to this plane of existence. We then intentionally caused each part of ourselves to forget our true nature and incarnate here at various levels of awareness with various physical forms such as people, plants and minerals, so that we could have the tremendous experience of awakening, remembering and returning to our true reality. Why would we do this? If who we are is love and joy, peace and wisdom, and there exists no opposite to this, how can we fully appreciate it? If all that exists is beautiful, how can we know it is beautiful? A great quote to summarize this concept is, "In the absence of that which we are not; that which we are is not." That is the answer, and that is why. (You may need to pause, re-read and reflect on this statement for a moment.) This means that in order to know oneself as something, the opposite to that must exist. It's all about relativity and duality. If I am all knowledge and love, I cannot fully appreciate it unless I experience myself as ignorant and selfish, at least temporarily. We have created the grandest drama of creativity, a 4-D holographic illusion full of experience, activity, and emotion. When we get tired of the show, we can always return to our infinite peace. If all this is true, how could we be assured that we will return to our true state of being after subjecting ourselves to this illusory creation? The genius of the design seems to be the law of karma. Since we have the innate sense of attraction and repulsion, we naturally learn to avoid causing suffering. Through the law of cause and effect, we learn from our experience what causes our suffering and how to avoid it. Ultimately, we find that seeking joy through outward means is the root of all suffering; we eventually realize that we must search within. We realize that if we don't go within, with true happiness we are without. Thus, with guidance and practice we succeed; our return is hence assured. Knowing this relieves us of fear. All fear stems from the fear of death. Realizing that we never truly die, but only change our frequencies and bodies, we feel truly free. You may find this perspective to be a higher consciousness, which enables you live with increased peace and happiness. Realizing the turmoil of this world to be ultimately an illusion frees you. Since all our suffering is temporary, we will eventually awaken from this awake-dream permanently. If we want to return to our source faster than living out the sequence of karma for many more lives, then perhaps we can practice the methods mentioned previously and to be introduced shortly. If we do not feel ready, we can at least live life as though we were already there. "Be the peace you would like to see in the world." Do the best you can to be balanced, disciplined, healthy, peaceful, creative, and loving to everyone. Doing this will bring instant happiness to yourself and others.

Is the process of creation expounded upon here actually true? How can all these things be stated so authoritatively? Perhaps they are intuitive revelations, which seem reasonable and logical, and the author presumes them to be true. Perhaps other explanations revealed to the author have been proven, and thus the accuracy of other statements received from the same source, are also inferred. Whether or not you choose to accept these statements as true for you, is your choice. If you are not yet sure and require further information, don't worry, this book isn't finished yet. Remember, the truth should be something that you can prove to yourself, not just take the word of another. If the ideas presented here are applied and found to be useful, then they are true for you. If not, perhaps they are true but you didn't really apply yourself. If that is so, then it simply wasn't the time for you now or the proper format, but you will eventually be led to the right circumstances. Maybe you will have applied the ideas here and found them to be useless, in which case their being untrue has become true for you. Thus, they will have still led you to the truth. Essentially there is no true right or wrong in the world of duality, everything is relative. The world's view on right and wrong is constantly changing as we evolve. In addition, even during a given point in that evolution, not all agree on what constitutes right and wrong. Take the topics of homosexuality or abortion, for example. These are constantly debated subjects. So whatever we do define as true for us comes down to what works for us at the time. It is not wrong to intend to drive to New York, but follow a route which leads to Miami instead. But since your intention was to go to New York, it didn't serve you to go to Miami. Therefore, we may say it's healthy to be vegetarian, but if someone has been vegetarian for 10 years and then one day has a hamburger, is that wrong? No, but given their intentions it may not have served them to give in to the impulse. One burger after 10 years will probably do no harm; however, it may have caused the person eating it to have less will-power. It may have contributed in a small way to slaughter of animals or been a bacteria laden piece of meat causing the person to become ill. But does that mean it was inherently wrong? Is there an unpleased Spirit; is this person to be punished? I think not. The point is that everything is a choice. We can observe the results of our choices and then decide what it means to us, thus affecting further choices. Thanks to our memory we can remember similar choices of the past and avoid what we may consider mistakes in the future. But that doesn't mean what did or did not work in the past will or will not work in the future. Since we are always changing, so is our individual perspective on what works for us. You may have decided that eating meat is healthy and that you need it for protein. You may have also decided that working out to get big muscles is the way to go, and anyone that didn't agree is weak. You may have decided that it's fun to mock vegetarians. But then one day, perhaps you changed your attitude. Maybe you realized that working out is good for being healthy, but trying to have big muscles alone is compensation for insecurity. Perhaps you became aware of alternative sources of protein such as soy and realized that years of eating meat collects toxins in the body which later manifest as disease. Maybe, awareness of the laws of karma developed and it was decided that it's not nice to mock vegetarians. Maybe you even became one. Society as a whole changes its collective mind as well. Fashion is considered hip in one generation, then out of style in the next, only to come back a generation later as retro. Also, what we consider acceptable is evident in the media. Twenty years ago, no one was singing about violence and drugs. Based upon observations, promoting excessive violence and negativity in movies, music, and video games seems to have affected our youth resulting in school shootings, and increased violence in general. It seems to rise in proportion to the levels of content that we condone. If what we say we want is a peaceful and safe world, then our choices are obviously not serving us. Perhaps we should choose to change what we deliver to the public. The media will tell you they are only supplying what the people want, but if that were the case, there wouldn't be any TV commercials, right? I don't think we want those. They are trying to sell us things. We can't control what they do, but we can control what we do with our choices. If we stopped buying what they are selling, we stop supporting it; then they are forced to come up with something else. If we stop buying meat, they will stop killing animals. If we stop buying into and watching violence, maybe we will stop doing it. Or, conversely, are we are into violence because we are violent by nature? Which came first, the chicken or the egg? If we are violent, and that is what we want to be, is it then wrong to be violent? The answer is not necessarily to try to stop everyone we disagree with, but we can stop watching or listening to them. We can educate others to do the same. Then one day, society chooses differently and what we were opposed to becomes obsolete anyway. The problem is that not all of us agree on what we want. That brings us to an amendment to the idea of it all being about choices. That amendment is acceptance. This is actually the secret of detachment. We make choices and carry out actions to manifest our choices. Yet, we may be going against others who are making opposing choices. Thus, if we want to not become angry or unhappy in life, it seems that the wise (second) choice would be to accept the reality of the present moment. This is what is referred to as being in the now, or simply being. Maybe we can't all have everything our way all of the time. Not trying at all isn't the answer. Trying and expecting exact results every time isn't realistic either. Therefore, the balanced perspective seems to be to try without being attached to certain expectations, and then accept the result of our actions. If we are not pleased with the result, we can always try again. Once we experience the result we intended, how do we feel about it? Did it serve us? Are we satisfied with our choice? Did our choices fulfill our expectations? If not, we may change our choices. Even if we are satisfied, we may end up changing our minds in the future during similar circumstances. This means that when we encounter someone else with an opposite view point to ours, in order to avoid negative feelings regarding that individual, we would be wise to remember that another person's choices (which we consider wrong), are our own choices of the past. That is the nature of forgiveness. Why are we discussing this? Because one thing most of us agree on is that people want peace. However, most people are unaware that their own choices are what cause their own perceived non-peace. Bringing to light observations of the nature of people's choices based upon the transitory nature of right and wrong, and the consequences of these perceptions enables us to become equipped with the power to make other decisions, such as what we want to feel and experience as a result. This is the power of true adaptability which we have been describing with the words: choose, detach, accept, and forgive. When practiced these words bring us peace. This is because the ultimate decision we can make is what we choose to be in relation to everything else that exists or occurs. Will we choose to try this for ourselves? Is peace something we talk about, something we believe in, something that we choose, or is peace something that we decide to be?

Chapter 3

We have been exploring the concept of love and peace as being the truth and reality of who we are. We have examined the practicality and even the necessity of incorporating these traits into our lives. Although this may work with results you can experience right away, we have also been mentioning methods to go deeper within, to bring about a greater awareness, higher consciousness, and results which are sustained more consistently and eventually, indefinitely. That is because there are many levels to our being. These parts of our being, (which are body, mind and Soul), do not always agree. That is why a discipline of practicing actual methods to become externally inactive and looking within is also necessary in order to re-establish balance and experience true freedom. The methods of yoga being referred to are an ancient, universal practice of developing balance, physical purification, spiritual devotion, and mental concentration used to begin true meditation; Although ancient, completely relevant and perhaps essential to sustaining modern humanity. This practice is the substance that seems lacking in religion today. Meditation, the most important part of the yoga system, (but can be utilized independently of it), is concentration used to realize the Soul; and the Soul is a part of Spirit. It is the ultimate unification. This state is what is known as, Enlightenment, God-Realization, or Self-Realization. The process of yoga ultimately culminates with a joyous union of Soul and Spirit, like a glass of water poured into the ocean. Our ego-mind and body are the glass, which causes the separation consciousness, our Soul is the water in that glass, and the ocean represents the Spirit which we feel separate from. Of course, we are not really separate, but just experiencing that we are. Yoga is believed to be a proven system to obtain everlasting freedom and happiness by facilitating the experience of going beyond the body, and mind to realize the Soul. Yoga is available to all regardless of social and financial status or religion. It is being presented for you here stripped of any theological ideology. You will find no preaching here, only effective methods extracted, organized, explained and presented in a contemporary manner for your study and experimentation. Do not be fooled by impressive words. The techniques themselves are so simple that unless the purpose and theory are understood, there is risk that they may be disregarded. The ego loves complexity. That is how it enslaves us to perpetually think. By doing so, we are erroneously convinced of getting nearer to the truth when in fact we are just going in circles. The only way to reach the source of those thoughts is to transcend the mind. If we can do that, it is natural to assume that by becoming one with the source of all knowledge, there would no longer be a need to ascertain knowledge by thinking. Hence, the way to do this is actually very simple, but the practice of it will contradict the current habits of extreme activity so much, that it may be the most difficult thing you ever attempted. Do not be discouraged, because it may also be the most important thing to do. It is interesting that with yoga and/or meditation, the intention is that practice literally makes perfect. Although the actual techniques will be revealed later, let's take a sneak-peek at what's to come. In order to still the mind and body and become sensitive to the finer details of being, the most significant tool we can utilize to become relaxed, quiet and concentrated is to focus on the breath. You may have begun to realize this from the Detachment meditation from Chapter One. A person eventually realizes that the person he/she thought they were was only a wave of ego on the oceanic consciousness of the omnipresent, omniscient Spirit. That really a part of this became many reflections of itself, reflections that forgot their true origin due to ignorance, desire, fear and aggression. Subjected to a cycle of cause and effect, the ego became deluded and fell into the habit of believing that it (the reflection) is the true identity of the Self. If we want eternal happiness, we must learn to re-associate our consciousness from the ego-mind and body, to the Soul; and then unify our Soul with Spirit. We quite literally need to go, out of our mind, and return to our source. But how can we accomplish this? Discipline, will power, study, practice and patience are all that are required. We all possess these traits only most of us do not utilize them in the most beneficial manner or to the appropriate degree.

In this book some Sanskrit terms are used to define certain aspects and processes. The methods of yoga originated where Sanskrit was the language used at the time. It is believed that Sanskrit, which has an alphabet of fifty letters or symbols, is the foundation of all language in the world today. It has also been described as "perfect," or nearly so. Unlike many other religious texts believed to have been inspired by the Divine, the Sanskrit texts have remained remarkably unchanged since their creation. This is because they were not translated hundreds of times, or edited/censored for political or other purposes. They are still in the original language for those that understand it, but have also been translated to English in this century. The most important and relevant works, (to the author), whether scripture or not, are listed in the Bibliography of this book; but there are also many other scriptures considered important as well, to many people that are not listed. In the quest for truth, it is natural to act as an investigator and scientist. First we look for clues, then we back-track to find the source of our information. This is followed by careful research of the evidence and careful application. Judging from the results, we decide if the revealed truth works for us or not. If not, we discard it; if so, we continue our efforts until we not only know the truth, but also become it. Sometimes this quest can become daunting and many people find it helpful to refer to literature such as this to remind them of the reason and maintain their motivation.

Certain principals of exactly how some schools of yoga teach that the Soul became encased within earthly matter and the process of reversing it will be explained at this time. The proclaimed yogis of the world from ages past have allegedly reached high spiritual planes and accessed certain information, which details the creation process for human life which has not yet been entirely corroborated by science in our Age. However, I believe you may find the following information logical and useful. Remember, that all that exists is energy at various frequencies, which due to our senses appear solid. Remember also that there exists the Unseen which is also likely to be just as real, yet invisible to us. Although we exist on one plane where objects are vibrating at relatively the same frequency, there are dimensions we do not perceive, but can potentially if we change our frequency.

The Sanskrit word for your Soul's concentrated energetic form is known by those who practice yoga as, the "Kundalini." It is said that the kundalini is the essence of your being and it enters this world based upon karmic and astrological factors at the moment when sperm unites with ovum. It then forms what later becomes the medulla oblongata located at the base of the skull. As the physical body is formed in the womb of the mother, the kundalini energy travels down within the spine leaving behind nerve centers called, "Chakras." These chakras correspond to certain specific aspects of the basic elements of nature and are also related to the five senses. As it travels downward, it finally reaches the tail of the spine and settles into a coil. One may bring the kundalini back up the spine and rejoin with the Source by living in harmony with nature and cultivating methods like yoga meditation to become balanced. Advanced teachings also state that by using the power of meditation, one may consciously circulate this energy around the chakras, thus hastening one's evolution. This is because the chakras are supposed to be related to the planets astrologically. Being a part of the whole, the blueprints for the universe are also within us. To reconnect to your higher self, would be the completion of your being. A re-association of your consciousness from the little, seemingly separate self you experience now, to the incredible infinite love and intelligence, which created it all, is to lose your false sense of self and attain the real one. An appropriate analogy would be like one of the blood cells in your body thinking it was the highest state of perception, until it somehow had the opportunity or ability to expand its sense of self beyond being a cell, into being your entire body and seeing out of your eyes as a total human. We are like the cells and Spirit is the complete body. Spirit encompasses all because it is the substance which creates and sustains all that is. You are not a human having a spiritual experience, you are a Soul/Spirit having a human experience; that is why we do not remember the larger self and it seems unreal to us. We have held onto this limited perspective for too long. It is fine to enjoy ourselves here, but if we become tired of the in-harmony, limitations and suffering, then it is time to raise our consciousness and return to our true nature. That is when we seek out methods to do so. Having done so, we practice a system such as yoga. After such practice we succeed in unifying ourselves once again. Repetition of this process is said to eventually allow us to maintain this state of awareness and being, indefinitely. You will find these statements repeated throughout the course of this book in order to enhance understanding and remembrance. If these ideas still seem strange to you, at least consider the possibility of their validity for now.

Some teachings purport that a seeker doesn't really need any sort of discipline to bring about a state of enlightenment. They state that Spirit's will (grace) is all that is needed, and that this can be brought on only by devotion only. But let us examine the validity of this concept. Each individual's life experience is unique and subject to an individual perspective. Thus, Reality may seem based on experience and hence, relative. Yet, the Reality we experience is limited in scope to our evolutionary development in linear time and will expand as our consciousness rises, and seem to have many levels; but in fact, the ultimate perspective is of the ones whom achieve the elevated state of being beyond the body, mind, intellect, ego, and emotions. The free state of being is no longer colored, or filtered by these personal traits of the ego-mind, and able to clearly experience the Reality in its entirety. It is this "true" perspective that is referred to as enlightenment; and from these that we occasionally receive guidance and refer to as intuition. This is a state of being, not a place, but rather a state inside you and what we call Spirit or the Higher-Self, or any name by any religion. It may be glimpsed from time to time based on various conditions or reasons. So in this way the previous statement about enlightenment being brought about without discipline is partially true. However, due to our unrefined nature, it probably cannot be maintained, (in the rare case that it was glimpsed at all); But by practicing the methods outlined in these pages, persons have purported to methodically refine themselves until a state of balance and purification was reached on all levels. When this happens and a high degree of concentration is cultivated and utilized, the highest state of being might be realized and maintained. It seems that if true, this should be the ultimate goal of all mankind, regardless of the temporary individual desires of each person's ego. This is a state of being that will be maintained even beyond the death of your body. You may need to reincarnate in order to fulfill certain karmic obligations, but once these are fulfilled, you will no longer return unless you wish to help others. Perhaps there are higher worlds for you to enjoy if you choose; or maybe at the highest level you will feel that you actually are the entire universe itself and no longer need to incarnate into a physical body. Rather than seeking joy, you will actually *be* the highest state of joy, which is what God is supposed to be; which by default makes you literally, exist within (be in) God; or you could say, being God, or even a God-being. Since that same joy-energy is in all life, this means you are one with all other things, with all of life. Everyone is you. We are one. If part of the reason of our existence is to realize this and align ourselves, thus discovering the love within, which is devotion, a love for Spirit; could grace be bestowed instead, (as some claim), negating a need to practice any methods? If that were the case, we need to question what would have caused that individual to have the ability to receive this (and not us) if they have been subjected to all the similar circumstances and are composed of all the same elements as us. It seems that it could only be due to the culmination of lessons learned over numerous lifetimes. The old masters say it takes about a million of these. That seems like a long time to suffer. Of course since we are all part of that eternal source, we are here to experience ourselves at different levels of our consciousness. This means there is no judgment, it's all about what we choose to experience. Do we choose to live against the natural laws of creation and suffer, or do we choose to discipline ourselves to realign with nature and experience our true beauty and magnitude? Do we choose love or fear? Do we choose to end the suffering? Well, most of us have not been around long enough to immediately have the experience of the "Spirit-Perspective," as I sometimes refer to it. That's why I believe that for most of us, the safest, surest route is to practice the methods of yoga, which includes meditation. You may ask, "...but what if this is unnecessary; and I practiced for nothing?" Well then, what will you have lost? You would have used just a little effort to live a life of balance and love, when you live eternally anyway. But what is the price of no effort; potentially, an unknown number of lifetimes in ignorance and suffering? I think the pros out way the cons here, but what do you think?

There are various branches of yoga, and different schools within of each of those branches. Hatha Yoga is very popular now as many have become aware of the fitness and health benefits of the postures that are practiced in this branch. Hatha is just one of the several branches of yoga. Of Hatha Yoga alone, there are many schools for each of the many styles that you can practice. It is possible to do a flowing routine of physical postures moving gracefully from one posture to another, and there are styles in which one works with only a few of them as a form of concentration. The other branches focus on chanting, breathing, or other methods. These branches will be broken down and explained shortly. It may take some study and experimentation before you settle on a particular path that you feel is most right for you. They all work, they all bring you to the goal, but since we each have different personalities, what works for someone else may not work well for you. The reason they all do work, however, is because the *core essence* of each of these teachings is the same. Each one leads you to eventually forget the ego, and increase concentration on the present moment, the present state of being. Each one will develop the discipline to literally choose a state of being for the present moment rather than be a victim of emotion and circumstance. The steps of yoga outlined apply to all yoga branches, but the various schools referred to, emphasize one part or another or focus on only certain parts. Practicing all of it and particularly the higher stages is known as, "Ashtanga" or "Raja" (Royal) Yoga. This is an elaborate, complete, logical and balanced system. As many people study and practice this, they begin to have many questions. These are often answered through intuition, directly in meditation, or through writing in a journal, a dream, being led to read something, or to talk to someone. The answers found inevitably lead to still other questions. One big question for me personally, eluded me for some time. As much as I felt I understood the process of yoga, I felt there was a part that I still didn't fully grasp. I understood that these methods, when practiced wholeheartedly and routinely, are thought to bring about a state of enlightenment known as, "Samadhi." I also knew that there was eventually the (supposed) rising of the kundalini force through the chakras; but I couldn't understand what the connection was between these two seemingly separate processes. I wondered, "If the Truth is realized through Samadhi, what is the correlation to the kundalini? Should it rise of its own accord or be manipulated, and what is the connection between the two?" I will convey to you now, what I perceived as the answer. By practicing yoga, especially meditation and the higher stages, we become balanced and purified, able to fully receive the intense power of the universe. Higher levels of consciousness are realized, but what I missed before was that the process of becoming balanced and purified is supposedly a direct result of the chakras being opened by the kundalini rising; That this was a simultaneous process, according to the sages. One starts by trying to cultivate only good karma by thinking, speaking and doing only positive things. This begins the purification. Purified due in part to our guiltlessness caused by living a life in tune with nature. Proper exercise or the Hatha Yoga positions bring physical balance and relaxation; they also may affect the chakras, (assuming chakras exist). The significance of these energy centers will be discussed in depth later. Proper breathing including the practice of controlled breath, known as "Pranayama," balances and relaxes the energy body, also called the "Astral" body and steadies the mind. Then one is prepared for the practice of concentration. One begins to detach from the bombardment of the senses, which in turn were generating distracting thoughts. Being thus detached, one is able to begin concentration. This is done until it becomes so deep, that eventually there are no thoughts other than of the object being concentrated upon. This frees you from your ego, thoughts and emotions. Being freed from who we thought we were, we are able to experience what we really are. But this brings us back to my original question. Although we may be able to get to this point of realizing the truth of who we are thus becoming enlightened and reaching Samadhi, due to the strong karmic pull of the world and our evolutionary state, we will not be able to maintain this awareness, this state of being. Which means the kundalini, (our consciousness and the concentrated energy of our Soul), will rise and connect us to our higher self, but will begin to drop back down the spine again. If a doctor gave a clinically obese patient liposuction, unless the patient changed their lifestyle habits they would eventually become obese again; the only difference is that the problem for the patient pertains to the future, where as the problem for us is in the past. You may have changed your attitude and lifestyle for the good now and for the future, but you may still have unfulfilled karmic obligations of the past. That is why we may need to meditate and make the connection again and again until we have burned off all the past karma and can maintain the kundalini at the high level and maintain the Samadhi state at all times. When this finally occurs one becomes known as an "Avatar," as were the historical figures of Jesus, Krishna and Buddha believed to be. So that is the answer to the question of what the connection is between enlightenment and the kundalini force rising. The kundalini rising is supposed to balance the chakras, preparing one for deep concentration, which unifies one with the higher-self. The repeated process of practicing should eventually enable one to maintain this state permanently. Thus permanent happiness is achieved; permanent since independent of the temporary conditions of this world. It is permanent and changeless and therefore, Reality. This ultimate state of being is like the third phase we spoke of earlier, the unconscious deep sleep state, except it is no longer unconscious but fully conscious; it now becomes a permanent return to your source of being, rather than a temporary nightly one. You could now maintain a state of aware being, beyond the three stages, and the mystery is solved.

Obviously, you are aware of the physical aspect of your constitution in this world, the body with its skin, bones, organs, brain, and so on. As explained earlier, everything consists of energy. This energy moves so fast that it appears to be solid and stable. Just as an ice cube seems to be so, yet when subjected to a change in conditions, that same form of a cube can change. If heated the cube shape of ice will melt into a puddle. If the puddle is excessively heated it will evaporate into the air. When the air becomes too saturated it will rain. The raindrops appear separate as individual drops but accumulate once again into one puddle. That puddle can be refrozen and reshaped, but through all these changes, the molecular constitution remains the same, H20. Samples were taken from the moon and they discovered the very same elements and minerals are there as we have here. Minerals and chemical elements found in nature are in your food, we need them because they are a part of us. We even take vitamin supplements. The point is that there are minuscule actions happening that we do not pay attention to, but exist and are a reality nevertheless. As pointed out earlier, these actions must be preceded by thought in order for all this organized activity to occur. Just ask yourself, "What causes us to breathe?" If you tried to stop, a very strong force would eventually compel you to take a breath, even if you succeeded in holding it for a long time. It is this same force operating which we don't understand because we don't pay attention to it. This force of energy, which has intelligence behind it, is the intelligence of our higher-self. So, as you have a physical body, you may know by now that you also have an energy body. As mentioned, this is referred to as the Astral body. You may have heard of some whom claim to be able to see this energy body, or you may have heard it described as having colors like a rainbow. It is also referred to as, your "Aura." In addition to the physical body and the astral body, there is believed to be the body of thought known as, the "Causal" body. You have your immortal Soul, encased in these three "bodies," the causal body of thought which causes the body of energy, which becomes solidified as the physical body. The five senses develop with the nervous system and the world attracts our attention, forcing us to experience it through our senses. This seems to go on for many incarnations and we become so intoxicated with the world that we begin to seek pleasure/happiness from it. We desperately extract it from new friends, goals, lovers, activities, and material objects. We eventually became disconnected from the higher part of ourselves, and have now reached a point in our civilization that we refer to that lost higher part of ourselves as a mysterious "God." Well fortunately, that higher part is wiser than us, (the lower nature), because there is a way out of this backwards mess. Just as there is a process underlying our creation, there is also a process to undo it and return to our origin. One such process is of course yoga. Don't be turned off by the terminology, yoga is not supposed to be a religion, although some schools have turned it into one. It is the science of returning to your true self, while leading a balanced and harmonious life with awareness. Yoga consists of techniques which together seem complex, but hypothetically someone could be practicing these methods while not even knowing they are practicing, "yoga." Some prefer only to practice meditation, which is the higher part of yoga. That is fine also, but the entire system of yoga is designed to foster a balanced life and facilitate an easier practice of meditation. Since I not only encourage the practice of meditation as a part of the yoga system, but also want to emphasize the importance of meditation, I refer to the methods outlined in these pages as, "Yoga Meditation," rather than yoga *and* meditation. It doesn't matter what we call it, these are actual, methodic ways to ease suffering, increase empowerment, actively participate in creation, and to find a greater and more sustained happiness than was thought possible. Let's move on to explaining this process and its correspondence to existence.

Compiled by the sage, Patanjali Maharishi, in the "Yoga Sutras," the "Eight Limbs" (of Yoga) are a complete series of methods outlining how to balance and purify the body and mind, ultimately transcending them, and leading one to spiritual enlightenment.

THE EIGHT LIMBS OF YOGA

1. **Yamas** - The Yamas or restraints (Don'ts) are divided into five injunctions. They should be practiced in thought, word, and deed:
    - **Ahimsa** - non-violence.
    - **Satyam** – truthfulness.
    - **Brahmacharya** - moderation in all things, control of the senses.
    - **Asteya** - non-stealing.
    - **Aparigraha** - non-covetousness, non-desire.

2. **Niyamas** - The Niyamas or observances (Do's) are also divided into five ethical precepts:
    - **Saucha** – purity, internal and external cleanliness.
    - **Santosha** – contentment, detachment.
    - **Tapas** – austerity, simplicity.
    - **Swadhyaya** - study of the spiritual texts.
    - **Ishwara Pranidhana** - constantly living with an awareness of the Divine Presence.

These 10 attributes fall under the category of "Discipline & Detachment." (Please refer to the **Freedom Formula** found on page 38.) If one were detached, there would be no desire and therefore no violence, lying, or stealing because there would be no need for things to be any other than they are already, and to be this way implies you are also aware. If one were disciplined there would naturally be moderation, cleanliness, simplicity, detachment and study. These Yama/Niyamas may seem a bit repetitive, but I believe this was intended to outline a positive and negative portrayal of each quality.

3. **Asanas**- Posture(s). A Regulation or control of the **body**. One of the reasons for the postures is the necessity of maintaining the body in a steady and still posture as preparation for the next steps. Therefore, a certain series of postures are performed in conjunction with the next phase of breath regulation. Performing a series of asanas is known as Hatha Yoga.

4. **Pranayama**- Regulation or control of the **breath**. Breath connects body to mind and is also a form of energy. By bringing the breath under control and relaxing it, we are able to relax the mind.

5. **Pratyahara**- Withdrawal of the senses in order to still the mind. By bringing the body, breath and mind into a relaxed state, we become aware of the breath becoming increasingly refined until we notice the foundation of Prana or energy in

the spine. As we focus on that, the senses are withdrawn. Essentially, this can be considered a regulation or control of the **senses**.

6. **Dharana**- Concentration. Regulation or control of the **mind**. Since relaxation of body, breath, mind and the senses has occurred; the mind is able to focus without distraction until it gradually merges into the next phase. The object of meditation selected may begin as an external one such as, a candle flame, but will eventually become internal such as, the sacred energetic sound of "Om," which permeates all existence and becomes increasingly apparent. (Om is explained further on page 105.) Or, perhaps the object may even be the flow of prana (energy) such as the kundalini in the spine. (The eyes are supposed to be gently gazing at the "spiritual-eye" between the eyebrows, but you may choose not to.)

7. **Dhyana**- Meditation. This is the next phase where concentration has become so deep and intense, that the state of one pure thought and absorption in the object of meditation has been achieved. (There is still duality in Dhyana.) The kundalini is said to rise in the spine toward the spiritual eye, activating the chakras. This becomes a regulation or control of the **energy** of your being.

8. <u>**Samadhi**</u>- The super-conscious state of non-duality of subject and object are experienced. Samadhi is the deepest and highest state of consciousness where body and mind have been fully transcended, and the Yogi finally experiences oneness with the highest and truest God-Self; the ultimate object of meditation. (Repeated contact with this state is supposed to be necessary for one to overcome karma and maintain this permanently and without further effort.) This mastery can be considered a regulation or control of the **Soul/Spirit**.

* * *

"Shutting out all external sense objects, keeping the eyes and vision concentrated between the two eyebrows, suspending the inward and outward breaths within the nostrils and thus controlling the mind, senses and intelligence; the transcendentalist aiming at liberation becomes free from desire, fear and anger. One who is always in this state is certainly permanently liberated." – The Bhagavad Gita.

* * *

Hopefully you have already realized the importance of the first two limbs of yoga, the **Yamas** and **Niyamas,** (do's and don'ts). Adhering to these are not rules to limit your freedom, they are more like suggestions or guidelines designed to expand you; though to the unrefined ego they seem more like limitations because the ego has not yet been disciplined. But following these precepts frees you because it assists in undoing the ignorance we suffer from. The ignorance defined is the ignoring of the truth. The truth is that we are one. What you do to another, you do to yourself. By following these two precepts we put ourselves in harmony with the truth and thus no longer have a subconscious, self-destructive feeling of guilt, which actually blocks our love and happiness. This generates peace and makes possible the deeper study of yoga.

The third step is the **Asana**, which is the correct posture. Sitting in correct posture is to sit with the spine straight. You do not lean against the back of the chair. Your feet are flat on the floor. Your hips are to be higher than your thighs. You may need to experiment with cushions to get the right position. You also may sit in the lotus posture (pg. 83), if you are flexible enough, or just cross-legged. Your head looks forward, straight ahead. The point is to make sure you sit straight, comfortable, aligned, alert and relaxed. The magnetic pull of the Earth is marginally counterproductive, but it is believed that placing a wool blanket underneath you aids in muting the force. Facing north or east is also supposed to help. You may also find it beneficial to practice Hatha Yoga. This develops the discipline necessary to sit in your Asana for prolonged periods of time, which is necessary to achieve the peaceful stillness required for the next steps. There are other benefits that will be discussed in greater detail as we proceed. This leads us to the fourth step **Pranayama**, which naturally follows from the previous three.

First of all, you should know that the mind and the breath are actually connected. Secondly, that we suffer from our ignorance due to the constant fluctuations of our mind's thoughts between desire and aversion, between the past and the future. If you think about it, all our complex thoughts come down to these simple states. We spend our mental energy either reminiscing our past achievements and pain experienced, or we contemplate the future with desire, what we hope to have and achieve, or avoid or destroy. Then we have the breath, which relentlessly passes through us during life, without stopping. Of course you are used to this, but it's like living with a radio which has a lot of static, if that is all you ever had, you will be used to it, and not know anything better exists. But because the mind and breath are connected, the mind never really has peace unless the breath stops.

Now it will be shown how the breath is connected to the mind. Due to thoughts, you have the breath. But because you are breathing, you are not relaxing as deeply as you could be. So, many ages ago, pundits discovered that by controlling your breath, you could control your mind. You don't have to understand this to believe it, just try it for yourself and you will see. So your breath swings back and forth, and your thoughts jump from past to future. These thoughts create emotional reactions to the thoughts, further complicating matters. There are different combinations of controlled breathing ratios to put an end to this. The easiest is to begin slowly inhaling and allowing the air touch the back of your throat. You may find yourself able to expand the inner throat a little, which allows you to feel the breath as a cool menthol-like sensation. It is ok if this is not felt right away, but with a little practice it should become natural. As you breathe in, count mentally until the lungs are full, this may be a count of 10 or 20, etc. Then, begin to exhale to the same count. This will force your breath to become even and stable. It will also calm it and your mind. Any emotions you are experiencing will temporarily subside. After repeating this perhaps 12 times or so, one stops and releases to simply observe the breath. You observe it in a detached way as though you were watching someone else breathing. This helps you to disconnect from the false idea of who you are and prepares you to receive the full truth. More specifically you will see that the longer you are able to sit motionless, ignoring the impulse to adjust too much or scratch or be otherwise distracted, the more you will find your breath to settle. You will also find that the breath is seemingly able to relax infinitely further. You can even imagine how it could become calm enough to stop altogether. Think of this like a pendulum which swings to and fro, becoming slower and slower until it eventually ceases. There will be spaces between your thoughts. Focus on the stillness between them, do not be afraid. The previous steps helped to balance the physical body, but this step balances the mental and astral. The connection between the mind and breath is the energy of the astral body. In some practices, Pranayama can be used to go beyond the simple counting stage to a visualization of the kundalini revolving around the spine. As concentration develops, this purportedly becomes less an exercise in visualization and more a reality of control, not only the breath, but of the energy itself. Did you ever notice that when you are concentrating on some thought or activity, your breath stops momentarily? Well it stops longer during higher stages of Yoga Meditation because breathing isn't necessary as much in that state. Remember, when you are in a state of being the energy, you do not need to extract it from sources outside of yourself. More specifically, you are so relaxed at that point that your body no longer needs to pump blood with the heart to oxidize the venous blood. Therefore, breath is not all that necessary either. The heart may even actually stop for a time. You are literally practicing entering the mysterious state of death. You will be realizing that "breathlessness is deathlessness." You are like a glass of liquid with debris inside. Can you sit still long enough for the liquid to settle and the water to become clear? If you can, you may experience the simple truth of your eternal nature which can never be destroyed: Existence, Consciousness, and Bliss.

The result of this practice leads to the next stage, **Pratyahara**. This is when the senses which have been causing you to be distracted by this world and disrupting your concentration, begin to reverse. Rather than flowing outward they flow inwardly. By concentrating on your breath and deepening your relaxation, your mind becomes fit for concentration. But true deep concentration can only occur if the senses are essentially turned off. Fortunately, this occurs simultaneously with Pranayama and the beginning of **Dharana**, the practice of concentration. But when the senses no longer disturb your practice, this becomes **Dhyana**, or Meditation. First we attempt to concentrate on an object or the breath, or a sound such as **Om**, the original causal vibration of our universe. At first the yogi and the object of meditation are separate, but eventually they become one. When this happens, we actually transcend not only the body, but also (finally) the mind. When we can transcend our mind, we can experience our Spirit. By bringing the body under control and disciplining it to be still, we can let go of it and focus on the mind. But to calm the mind, we need to discipline and control the breath. By doing this, the mind becomes calm. When the mind is calm, the senses and thoughts subside. When they subside, true concentration becomes possible. When deep concentration develops and intensifies, subject and object unite. When this occurs, the mind and ego are transcended and the lower nature and higher self unite. This is the final stage known as **Samadhi**. As mentioned earlier, this is a temporary but conscious return, but may become permanent with repeated practice. It is said that eventually we should feel at one with everything at all times, feeling all things to be an extension of ourselves. The only thing real is love. We will not resist situations and circumstances, understanding them to be part of the show and plan. We will accept and forgive the negativity in the world, realizing that without it we would be unable to experience being the opposite of that.

Think of our physical body as a guitar. The astral centers (chakras) along our spine are like strings of the guitar. We have been like guitars which are out of tune. Our mind can be the tuning device. The act of concentration is to tune the guitar; (becoming balanced). Our Soul represents the musician who plays the guitar, which is our body. The Spirit is the music itself. It is the musician's responsibility to keep the instrument in tune. However, as musicians, we have neglected our duty and denied we even have one. Due to this ignorance, we have been creating music which is out of tune and unbearable to listen to. If we each cultivate and use our concentration, our chakras (the strings), become in tune and the instruments (each other), become in harmony. Thus, we begin to make beautiful music together, and the world is a better place to live in, (listen to). We are literally Spirit's instruments, but we may also choose to elevate our perspective to that of the music itself. (Unite with the higher-self.) Any musician will concur that their best moments have been when they were able to forget themselves for the moment and become one with the music. So, Spirit is the music, the yoga system is the music instructor, your Soul is the musician, your body is the instrument, your mind is the tuner, your energy and chakras are the notes which need to become balanced by being in tune, and the world is the music we create. We should guide our music with discipline and wisdom and not indulge in playing reckless, inharmonious notes, since we have to listen to what we create, (cause and effect karma). We are the great orchestra, and we must *conduct* ourselves accordingly if we really want to live in peace.

* * *

As we learn to balance our body and mind, we develop the ability to control our energy.

As we learn to detach from our body and mind, we release the power of Spirit.

As we learn to tune in with Spirit, our consciousness expands to include everything else as an extension of itself.

Our domain of energy control is thus expanded beyond our body and mind, and extended into all that is.

Since all that exists is composed of energy, and all energy is Life, we become empowered to not only live our life, but to own it. Not just experience, but create it.

* * *

Chapter 4

This chapter will serve as a review, elaboration and clarification on the topic of yoga. This will be achieved by simplifying the concepts down to a core essence, which will deepen one's understanding of the process.

As we have discussed, this is a world of matter. Matter consists of energy. The illusory bridge between who you think you are and who you actually are (Spirit) is a matter of varying frequencies of energy, (rates of vibration). As you are already aware, our perception of reality is limited by our constitutional energy frequency. It has been stated here that by practicing the methods outlined previously, it is believed that one is able to raise that frequency thus experiencing and controlling higher states of energy, and therefore elevated states of consciousness, (since consciousness is refined energy). The highest state of energy would be the source of that energy, and that source is inferred to be Spirit. Accordingly, through utilizing a balance of discipline, detachment, devotion/love, awareness and concentration leading to meditation, we can reconnect with that source. As we engage in this process, it may be useful to have a deeper understanding of what may be encountered, and of exactly what occurs within us. This information, just as the previous, comes from those who have (presumably) followed the discipline of yoga to very high levels, and documented their knowledge for our benefit, much like an explorer. Most vibrations are occurring at speeds we cannot perceive with our senses directly, yet we know must exist because we have instruments which can detect this. Thus it is also safe to say there is still much more that we do not yet have instruments to detect, yet still also must exist. We know we have a physical body of course, because we can perceive it directly. We also know that there is an energy field behind everything, including the body. We stated that all thought precedes action, (energy is action), thus we infer the existence of intelligence under the energy body and refer to this as the mental or causal body, since it is the cause setting into motion the effect of the astral body, and subsequently the physical body. These are known as, "The Three Bodies." There are also the emotional and intellectual bodies, although they are not actually bodies per se, but with the above three can be collectively referred to as, "The Five Sheaths." At our core are also three fundamental and permanent traits, (not bodies or sheaths), "SAT, CHIT, and ANANDA." That is: Existence, Consciousness, & Bliss/Joy. Nothing can or will ever take that away. It is your eternal being.

Within the physical body there are obviously bones, muscle, organs and flesh. There are also a complex network of nerves and glands. Of course, you already know. What you may not know is that the connection of this physical system to the astral system. In Hinduism, Buddhism and mystical Kabbalah (among others), it is believed that the energy network of the astral body consists of chakras. These are believed to be like a bundle of nerves, except appearing as swirling, glowing lights. There are thought to be seven major chakras. In descending order they are as follows:

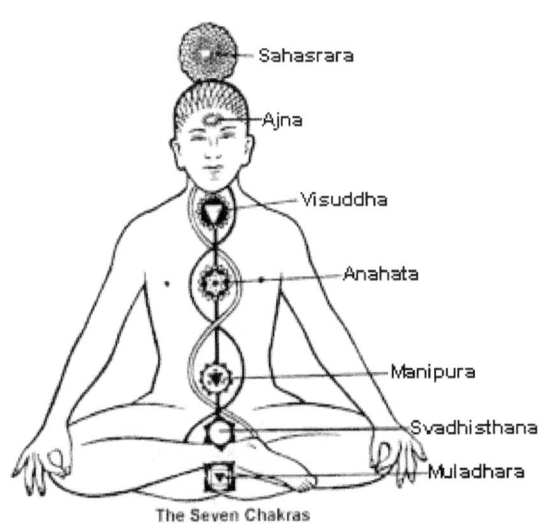

The Seven Chakras

THE CHAKRAS

7. _The Sahasrara Chakra_:
    - Located at the top of the head, near the brain. Crown.
    - Color is violet or even a golden white light.
    - Associated gland is the Pineal.
6. _The Ajna Chakra_:
    - Located in forehead, between the eyebrows. Cervical.
    - Color is indigo.
    - Associated gland is the Pituitary.
    - Also the seat of the spiritual eye or _Third Eye_.
5. _The Visuddhi Chakra_:
    - Located at the throat. Laryngeal.
    - Color is blue.
    - Associated gland is the Thyroid.
4. _The Anahata Chakra_:
    - Located at the chest, the heart center. Cardiac.
    - Color is green.
    - Associated gland is the Thymus.
3. _The Manipura Chakra_:
    - Located at the abdomen. Solar Plexus.
    - Color is yellow.
    - Associated gland is the Pancreas.
2. _The Svadhisthana Chakra_:
    - Located at the pelvis. Sacral.
    - Color is orange.
    - Associated glands are the Adrenals.
1. _The Muladhara Chakra_:
    - Located at the base of the spine. Coccygeal.
    - Color is red.
    - Associated glands are the Sex Organs.
    - Also the seat of the _Kundalini_.

*See the Appendix for more detailed information.

Chakras, Plexus, Glands & Nerves

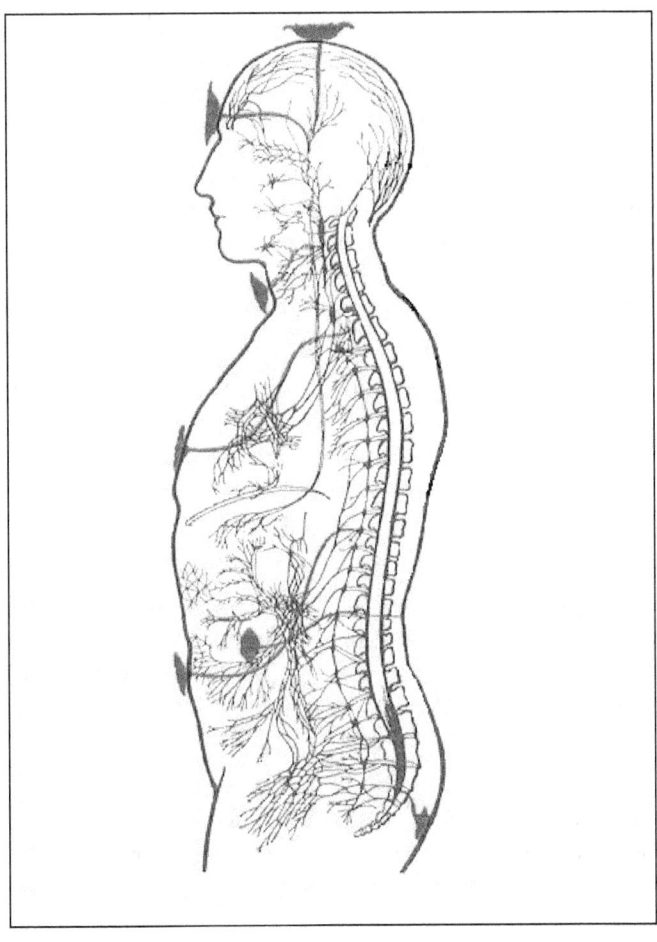

Depicted above, the glandular and nervous systems as is
believed to pertain to the chakras.

The chakras are described as being the spectrum of a rainbow. Any visual artist will tell you the colors mentioned here blend naturally from one to the other. Red becomes orange, orange becomes yellow, yellow becomes green, green changes to blue, blue changes to violet, violet becomes red to complete the circle, or in this case is the highest level and becomes golden or white. You will see that each of these chakras have an associated gland in the endocrine system which releases certain chemicals to the blood stream, and why learning to balance the chakras is believed to balance the body, mind and emotions. After reviewing the chart, you will have noticed that there are also corresponding sounds, (which are a variation of the original sound, Om), as well as associated musical notes which each resonates to, a particular crystal it responds to, a planet it is affected by (astrology), a specific associated scent, Sanskrit symbol, earth element, and personality trait. The chart visually depicts all of these attributes and their correlation to one another. Different spiritual groups and yoga schools disagree on minor points such as which specific planet may be related to a certain chakra, but this chart shows the most common consensus of how they all supposedly relate to the system of yoga as a process of balancing the entire being. In my opinion, these (chakras and forces described here) whether real or not, are not critical to the path, or our goal, but may be interesting speculation to learn what is taught by these schools. The chakra system and its correlation to the levels of our being seem convincing. If valid, we have the keys to unlock their potential. However, if they are not, then rest assured that any potential irrelevance does not negate or contradict the core essence of the yoga system (including meditation), which have been proven to be highly effective.

There are said to be ten types of, "Vital Force," which are the underlying forces of the more mundane processes of the body.

Major Forces:

1. PRANA = Heart = Respiration
2. APANA = Anus = Excretion
3. SAMANA = Navel = Digestion
4. UDANA = Throat = Swallowing
5. VYANDA = The Whole Body = Circulation

Minor Forces:

1. NAGA = Belching, Consciousness
2. KURMA = Eye lids, Vision
3. KRIKARA = Sneezing, Hunger, Thirst
4. DEVADATHA = Yawning
5. DHANANJAYA = Entire Body

- All of these Pranas are also governed by five "Vayus," or nerve currents.
- Related to the five senses: Smell, Taste, Touch, Hearing, and Sight.
- These are related to the five elements of Ether, Air, Gas, Fire, Water, and Earth.

Our states of existence are also said to be classified by the following three "Gunas," or states:

1. **SATWA** = Purity and knowledge, (positive)
2. **RAJAS** = Activity and motion, (neutral)
3. **TAMAS** = Inertia and laziness, (negative)

It is said that the subtle forces including the chakras govern the physical body. Yet it is also believed that these chakras can become imbalanced, resulting in disturbance to the entire being. Intertwined vertically through the chakras are, the "Nadis." The Ida and Pingali Nadis are said to look similar to a strand of DNA in structure and they carry the upward and downward currents of Prana (energy). When the chakras are balanced, the current is equal. There is also a Nadi in the center of the spine, passing straight through all the chakras. This is called, the "Sushumna Nadi." This is the nadi which the kundalini force allegedly travels upward through when released karmically or through yogic practices such as Hatha Yoga. This is because certain positions are supposed to be designed to force the body to send increased energy to a particular area. The system of Hatha Yoga includes a menu of postures for every part of the body, and therefore every known chakra. Other methods involve concentration on traits of the chakras such as their associated crystals, colors, sounds, or others listed in the chart.

The chakras are assumed to respond to this because thought is also a form of energy. Intense levels of will-power and concentration can send energy to certain parts of the body. Becoming balanced, they influence the mind, emotions and may also be responsible for affecting the body through the glands and other channels. One will know they are balanced when they feel steady peace, health, well-being, contentment, and high levels of creativity and energy. I'm not sure how much of the chart information is useful to the average person, or even to me, but I thought it would be best to include all information that I have acquired and leave it to the reader to decide what is, or is not important. This book contains some of the basic postures of Hatha Yoga in Chapter 8. If you feel the desire to learn more advanced postures, there are many other resources available. Some well-known and respected schools that produce books and/or videos on the subject include Sivananda Yoga-Vedanta Center, Iyengar Yoga, and Ananda. Through my research I believe I have been able to strip down to the bare essentials of all branches of yoga or any other practice with the same purpose of Self-Realization. There was a time when I was very absorbed in the complexity of various methods. At that point in my life I was not able to believe that a simple process could have the desired effect of Self-Realization. We always find what we believe we need to. Therefore, I did find schools that taught very detailed practices of visualization and concentration combined with many difficult postures and breathing exercises. Then I became aware that if one is able to understand the how and why of what yoga is doing, one becomes able to realize there is a certain simplified core essence that is common to all the programs. What has happened is that some of these various schools of yoga have become overly absorbed in the physical practice to the point of losing focus of the real goal. Perhaps in an age long ago, life was such that it was possible to spend half the day mastering various techniques. However in modern civilization, I find that for the average person there is not enough time to do so. Fortunately for us, I have also concluded that it is not necessary. But I have included much more information than I am currently utilizing for the reader to choose for themselves. Our perspective and needs are always changing; not only may I later decide or not decide to practice other techniques later for reasons I can not anticipate now, I am also aware that others reading this are at various stages of perception as well and may formulate their own practice including a combination of elements which I myself do not. That is why all the information is here. It's all about choice, right? But what I would like to accomplish is to have you understand the how and why, so that you are able to make a more educated decision about what you decide to practice. You will notice in the chart, that there are different yogas listed. These different branches emphasize various aspects of Patanjali's Yoga explained earlier.

BRANCHES OF YOGA

Hatha Yoga as you know, are the postures. We have already discussed the effect they have on the individual who practices the postures and how they are supposed to balance the chakras, and certainly increase flexibility, thus increasing the circulation of blood and energy to flow unobstructed throughout the system. It increases flexibility in the spine which it is believed leads to a longer and healthier life. It is also definitely a form of meditation in action as one becomes absorbed in the position, focusing inwardly on the body and breath, rather than the distractions of the outer world.

Karma Yoga focuses on "self-less" service, which means performing all actions without thought of the self. This is believed to help one learn to see others as themselves and do unto others as they would have done to them. This allows one to have a spiritual perspective because Spirit seems to serve all of life and need nothing in return. Humans usually act the opposite and therefore suffer. Karma Yoga helps one to reverse this habit. Most people feel good about doing this, but I believe you should make sure that no organization is taking advantage of your self-less service. If they do so, it is like you are subjecting yourself to voluntary slavery, and in my experience that does not help you to feel good about yourself. Yoga is supposed to be about feeling good. Karma Yoga also can be a meditation in action because when mastered, it enables one to maintain an elevated awareness throughout the activities of the day.

Mantra Yoga is the branch that emphasizes the chanting of certain words, phrases, or syllables that supposedly have high energy and positive impact when repeated due to the positive vibrations they produce. They are believed to have positive vibrations because they have certain root sounds, which are variations of the original causal creative vibration of Aum (Om); and because these same sounds have been presumably chanted for ages by highly evolved or enlightened beings. This sound represents the three stages of creation represented in the Hindu and Buddhist mythology by the Deity in three aspects of the creative, preserved, and destructive stages of life. All material creations go through these stages including us. Accepting this process of life helps us to overcome fear of death, and thus realize our spiritual immortality. We can learn to let go of our attachment to the physical and focus on the eternal part of our nature, which is the process itself. Chanting these vibrations or words which contain the same inherent meaning may raise one's consciousness because when one chants for some time, this becomes concentration. One becomes so absorbed in the sound of the mantra, that they can forget the ego self and instead experience the larger infinite Self. Thus it becomes a meditation.

Jnana Yoga is the yoga of the intellect. Some believe in the intense study and debate of texts that are considered scripture such as: The Bhagavad-Gita, The Tibetan Book of the Dead, The Upanishads, & The Yoga Sutras. Sincere study may allow one to expand their mind and elevate their consciousness. It is said that Buddha would sometimes teach one parable for the followers to meditate on for days until they became one with the concept, so this then can also be a meditation.

Bhakti Yoga practitioners believe that devotion alone is sufficient to attain Realization. They say that the intense love of Spirit and the Spirit in all raises the consciousness and energy including the kundalini. They also believe that a person's effort alone is not enough to attain the highest state, and that Spirit's grace is also required. By intense and sincere devotion, it is said that this grace can be received. (We have debated this view earlier.) Those who practice Bhakti may also include other aspects of yoga as a vehicle of reaching these levels of devotion. They may become full of love so deeply that they actually become one with it. If we have said that love is the essence of Spirit, then by becoming one with love, we can become one with Spirit. This then is also meditation.

Laya/Tantra Yoga is known for its sexual nature. "The Kama Sutra" is a popular book exploring the various sexual positions that may be used. True Tantra Yoga however is not solely for the purpose of sexual exploration. You will recall that yoga teaches in this world that there can be no pleasure without pain. That is why followers of yoga seek to overcome the karma cycle of suffering by learning to feel joy from within rather than feel transitory pleasure from the world, including sex. Sex is a very powerful force that has contributed to jealousy, desire and led to suffering. That is why celibacy is advocated in Patanjali's Sutras. The other reason is to conserve the highly creative and spiritual life force that is within the fluid secreted during this activity. In yoga, this force is related to the kundalini, the Soul's concentrated energy. That is why having sex can lead to a new life being born. Because in that fluid is literally the genetic and spiritual blueprint of life. It is truly a part of us participating in the creation of another. Of course, it is also a Soul that uses this as a vehicle to enter at conception. So this connection of sex to the kundalini is why it may be possible to raise the consciousness through sex. With this method the sexual fluid (and kundalini) may be controlled to move inward and up, rather than the common way of down and out. Most people are not capable of this kind of control, but I believe they may enjoy trying to through the practice of this yoga. In Tantra, the partners are supposed to see the Spirit in each other and use the act of sex as a way of harnessing the energy and connecting to their higher-selves. The intense love and attraction they have for each other is supposed to become so overwhelming that they first feel at one with each other, and then at one with Spirit. So you can see how this also is meditation.

Raja Yoga and in some traditions called Kriya Yoga, (although Kriya also refers to the practice of inner cleansing utilizing various techniques involving muscle control, breathing, cloth and salt water). Many yogis think of Raja as the highest or "royal" yoga because they believe that any one branch of yoga listed previously is not sufficient in itself. They believe that since balance is necessary in life for true harmony, then each branch of yoga is part of the whole system. Therefore they believe it is necessary to practice all parts of the system. Patanjali's yoga is classified as the Raja branch of yoga because it is a comprehensive, balanced approach that incorporates aspects of all the branches. The ethical precepts, physical postures, controlled (rhythmic) breathing, and detachment (via sense reversal), all combine to foster a culmination of meditator's consciousness unifying with the object of their concentration. This is the definition of true meditation and may also even eventually evolve into the highest stage, where the kundalini has risen and connected to the spiritual eye, and the consciousness temporarily leaves the body. In this stage one is supposed to be able to get a preview of death (in a positive way) by leaving the body and experiencing unity with the Spirit. In the complete mastery of yoga, this highest-self then "descends" in to the body and one becomes whole. They can then function from all levels of their being, in complete balance and supreme creative control. The goal of yoga is to be the tool to achieve this. Once at this stage, the tool no longer becomes necessary.

Kriya Yoga or **Kundalini** Yoga refers to a version of Raja Yoga practiced by members of a certain lineage of gurus from India ending with the last messenger of this line known as Paramhansa Yogananda. This teaching is Raja Yoga with the additional focus on an advanced stage of visualization involving the use of Pranayama and concentration on the kundalini energy in the spine, to not only consciously raise it, but also circulate it around the spine. Since the chakras may correspond to the planetary alignment of our conception and the astrological signs of the zodiac, it is believed that revolving this life energy around the spine is akin to hastening ones evolution and burning their seeds of karma. Rather than live out many more lifetimes, these yogis believe it is possible to essentially fast-forward their lives and achieve permanent return to Spirit in as short as one lifetime.

Any other names for yoga that you may have heard of are usually various schools a branch of yoga, such as Hatha Yoga. There are literally hundreds or even thousands of different Hatha Yoga schools. Each of these may not only teach the postures but also be influenced by a particular branch of yoga, or even a combination thereof. There are also numerous types of meditation such as, "Transcendentalism, (TM)." Like, Yoga, which Meditation is a part of, there is a core component of all schools or branches. As long as we know what it is, and how it works, it doesn't matter which version we use.

You can see how the point of all these branches of yoga and meditation is being in the present moment. Obviously there are many versions of what people believe is necessary from these branches and there are others also who have their own perspective on how what they consider necessary can be practiced. For example, in the practice of concentration, there are those who teach the discipline of detailed visualization of elaborate jewel encrusted rooms and spiritual guides. Then there are those who teach the practice of a simple concentration technique such as staring at a candle flame, or on the symbol of Om. Perhaps they disagree on technique, but if we are able to understand how and why meditation works, we can more easily distinguish what aspects we consider relevant and practical.

What I have discovered to be the *core essence* of all Yoga Meditation will be detailed now.

Physiology

The reason we suffer is due to the fact that our conscious awareness has been limited to body identification as slavery to the physical senses. As explained earlier, since we have this separatist mentality, we are in survival mode. We cater to the needs of the body. We seek satisfaction through outward means. Since the nature of the outer world is constant flux, the happiness we do receive is transitory, when that happiness has passed; suffering in various forms is experienced. This cycle repeats until we tire of it and seek a solution. We begin to discover that the answer is within. Meditation is the practice of doing so, of going within. Once we decide on a particular method of meditation, we should practice until we have mastered it. Not to do so is analogous to like we said earlier, trying repeatedly to get to a particular destination by driving one route only to turn back, start over and try another one. This is inefficient to say the least. We would never get where we intended to go. It is the same with yoga. We do not even have to label a system of going within as "yoga." There is an observable intelligent process in the workings of the body, the world and the universe; there are also definite methods of energy reversal from outward to inward focus. Do not be confused by the many branches, schools and methods. Essentially the process is deceptively simple but the intellect and ego believe that something as complex as life cannot have such as a simple answer. Yet the great irony is that often the best answer is the simplest one. The ego's purpose is to keep us confined to body identification, and fears its own death. It acts to keep us grounded in earthly pursuits much as gravity keeps us on the ground. If we were to personify this force, we may as well personify every known force including gravity. As a matter of fact, that is exactly what some societies have done. Many American Indians still believe there is a "Spirit" in everything. This is similar to the beliefs found in Greek mythology. But later in history, the majority of society agreed that there was essentially one Spirit. However, that doesn't mean that this (one) Spirit doesn't express its creative powers through Deities, (godlike entities, angels, saints or emissaries). Perhaps since everything is conscious energy at various levels of awareness, and all is living energy; then maybe they were not so far off after-all. Ultimately, there must be one source for all, and we are one with that source. So there is no need to focus on or fear any lesser Deity. Wouldn't the "Devil," if such a thing could even exist as some think of it, only be a manifestation of Spirit's idea and serving its purpose? Without the bad, there can be no good. I believe this devil figure is simply an ignorant explanation and personification of the force of ego and negative pole of the spectrum that we also refer to generally as, evil. Even if there are individual entities, good and bad, behind the operations of this world, are they not also from the same source, and therefore one with us? Would the positive and negative things which they cause to happen to us be any different than any other good and bad thing that happens? Wouldn't that still be the same law of karma in operation? We do not need to be concerned with this. When we master ourselves, we have mastered the universe and what then is there to fear? Fortunately the reality of the Spirit eventually overrides our ego and we begin to realize the possibility of separating from that which we have believed to have been us, and re-associate from the ego-personality to the true, eternal nature of the Spirit. Once we have done so, there can be no fear because as we have said, there is ultimately no death. We are energy, and energy cannot die.

Unfortunately, most religions have kept their followers ignorant of the truth by editing or mistranslating their sacred texts. They have used ignorance to keep their supporters controlled by guilt and fear. Most churches will talk to you about love and sin, but never explain the how and why of life or how we may free ourselves from the death-rebirth cycle. As we have covered under the section outlining Patanjali's yoga, there is Yama and Niyama, which are the guidelines that most or all major religions have in one form or another. The problem is that without an understanding, these become perceived as laws that are being dictated to us by an overlord that we must fear. However, with understanding, we realize that they are simply meant as a guide for us to realign ourselves with our true nature and thus cease suffering.

The ten Yama and Niyama precepts are hard to remember and keep in the forefront of the mind during day-to-day activities; and they can also be subject to misinterpretation. If you think about it, the core principals of these guidelines are that all others are an extension of yourself; Therefore, what you do to another you ultimately do to yourself, and that's how karma is believed to function. What goes around comes around;

this allows us to remember this fact of unity, through experiencing the effects of our actions. That is why we can sum up all these precepts with one familiar piece of advice: "Do unto others as you would have done unto you." The results of practicing this perfectly may be experienced immediately, or in linear time depending on your individual accumulation of karma for which there may be some that has yet to be fulfilled. Some also believe that even this karma can be overridden. Two ways to look at why it may be possible to override karma would be that:

1. There is the grace of Spirit, which may be pleased with your sincerity, spiritual effort, and progress. (That doesn't seem fair. As pointed out earlier, not everyone has equal opportunity in a particular life to acquire knowledge of yoga or similar methods of achieving liberation.)

2. We are one with Spirit because that is our higher-self. Since we are actively collaborating with the higher-self to create our reality, we can create the possibility of overriding our past karma. (We can be sure that we are one with Spirit, and even that we can affect our reality, but whether karma exists and can be over-ridden cannot be proven since we would have to have a memory of our past lives, if any.) So the simplistic aspect of the first and second limbs of yoga are to remember our essential oneness, and to think, speak and act with love for all-because that is what we should want in return for ourselves, if what we want is to be happy. It boils down to maintaining awareness through discipline and detachment.

The third limb is the Asana, but Patanjali doesn't specify Hatha Yoga. It is only stated that the purpose is to maintain a "steady pose." It is observed elsewhere that the practice of Hatha Yoga has many benefits which we have outlined previously and will continue with shortly. One of those benefits is that by mastering postures, one naturally also masters the central posture of sitting as preparation for meditation. Another reason Hatha is a benefit and is normally included with a school's yoga program is because practice of this branch of yoga develops stamina in the body, which conditions it with the ability to remain in a steady pose, comfortably, for long periods of time. If we do not exercise, the body stores too much energy and is more likely to feel compelled to act in the world, to do something. Also, by expending energy outwardly, you allow energy from the higher source to flow through you in order to recharge you. This is also what we can assume happens during sleep, or even when fasting. We reconnect to our source. If we see the practicality of including postures in our yoga, we may become daunted because we may feel there is not enough time for both practice of Hatha and meditation, which both require enough time for one to become absorbed and benefit thereby. That may be one reason why followers of Paramhansa Yogananda practice a 15 minute routine called the, "Energization Exercises." These are a series of physical movements intended to have the same benefits of Hatha Yoga, without the time or potential discomfort of certain postures. The postures are usually only uncomfortable when people have allowed their bodies to develop without stretching adequately throughout their life, thereby permitting the body to become stiff. Although yoga eventually allows one to regain flexibility, at first the body resists and is therefore uncomfortable. The reason this technique may be valid is because there is a simplistic core reason to how yoga works but we don't need to call it yoga or any other exotic word. So the point of the third limb is to exercise regularly. It doesn't have to be Hatha Yoga, but if you intend to meditate after, it is not wise to workout in a way that does not improve your spiritual awareness. Lifting weights to get bigger muscles is not necessarily wrong, but it may not be conducive to meditation as it is usually focused on aggression, body identification, and a high degree of stress. Of course, there are always exceptions to everything depending upon the consciousness of the individual. Personally, I recommend a practice of some basic postures such as the Sun Salutation. This is a series of 12 simple postures, which put the body in all the important positions. These can be done in half an hour or less if one chooses, before going into the other limbs of yoga. (See pgs. 141 – 145.)

The practice of Hatha Yoga involves the control of breath, (Pranayama). As said earlier, one is to perform the postures while paying attention to the rhythm of the breath. This aids in detaching from the body. While this calms the mind also, more importantly it is the bridge that prepares one to become aware of ever more refined stages such as of the source of breath, which is energy.

So the essence of this stage is to control the breath. It does not need to be complicated. Later we will see just how easy this can be.

The next limb is Pratyahara. This is inverting the flow of the senses by detachment. We have seen how only by disconnecting from our senses can we focus on the subtle movements within us. The various branches of yoga offer various techniques to do so. That is why they all work. But which one is suitable to your individual temperament is relative. The reason that it is debatable on if one branch alone is sufficient, is because it seems that each branch primarily affects only one aspect of our being. Since there are several levels to our being, it seems logical that there needs to be several aspects to our yoga practice. All branches are successful if they can enable one to detach from the senses and concentrate within. Some may find it easier to accomplish this through chanting mantras, some through performing postures. I find that detachment and the next stage of concentration can occur concurrently. As suggested earlier, although Patanjali's steps imply that detachment precedes concentration, I believe closer examination reveals that these are not strictly chronological steps as they are labels of major identifiable levels of a process which overlap and can occur simultaneously. For instance, we begin with moral conduct and physical postures, but we do not abandon these as we proceed to the other stages. That is why I have noticed that when we concentrate on something deeply enough, it seems possible to place your consciousness there. By doing so, haven't we transcended the senses? And so, it seems that detachment is something which happens as a result of the other stages but is not necessarily a step in of its self. It seems to be the result of deep concentration reached when practicing the other stages together, but particularly concentration. Although there does also seem to be a progression as one stage flows into the next as a process. One particular method of practicing detachment taught in this book is the "Om" (or "Hong Sau") technique whereby after one has succeeded in controlling the body and then breath, one attempts to let go of the breath rather than control it. Just as in Hatha Yoga there is tension followed by relaxation; here we have the same with breath, a control followed by a release. This release may assist one in disconnecting from the ego and body identification. It may occur because the body and mind have the breath in common. If we can disassociate from the breath, we also achieve separation from body and mind. In this technique one simply observes the breath as it moves in and out of the body. One observes in a detached frame of mind as though witnessing someone else breathing. In order to progress, once you are able to detach you must then inwardly focus your attention on something, rather than remain in a stagnant state of "no-mind."

Dharana or Concentration, as we know, is the deep attention to a specific outer or inner object. Mastery of this means one has unified themselves (the observer), the action of observation, and the object of concentration as one awareness. Hypothetically, if I concentrate on an apple long and deeply enough, I may be able to have the experience of being the apple temporarily. This occurrence is when concentration has become meditation. That does not mean that meditation is the highest stage. That is because meditation is the ability to have become one with the object of concentration. But clearly, becoming an apple is not the highest stage of this practice. Thus, logically we can conclude that if this is possible and we can change our object of concentration to the inner state, we must focus our concentration on an aspect of our energy instead. You can see how the stages of Patanjali's yoga actually do occur simultaneously, because concentration is necessary for many, if not all, of the 8 limbs (to some degree), especially from the 3rd to 8th limb. In Hatha Yoga we concentrate on the body and breath. In the next stage of Pranayama, we focus on the breath alone. This concentration on the breath allows us to detach and become aware of the inner energy field. We can then change our object of concentration from the body, to breath, to the energy. At that point we may not be aware of it, but we would have disconnected from the senses as we concentrated on the energy.

"OM"

This energy may become apparent as the Om vibration. All objects in this realm are composed of energy. The vibration of energy makes a sound, which permeates the entire universe. Om (pronounced "Aum") also represents the creative, preserved, and destructive aspects of nature. This creative vibration makes up "Maya" or the illusion of our physical existence. It is believed that one can reach higher states of consciousness and Self-Realization (with practice) by meditating upon or mentally chanting its sound. Om is the audible version of the infinite consciousness. Chanting "Om" may awaken your chakras because it is their origin and sustainer. As we concentrate on Om, we may become one with it. That is the beginning of meditation or Dhyana. Most people concentrate and say they are meditating, not realizing that true meditation is only happening when there is an actual unification. We then repeatedly practice meditation because there are progressively higher levels of awareness which can be experienced. Patanjali elaborates extensively on the numerous experiences encountered. So essentially we can practice a simple technique of concentration, which eventually becomes meditation. Once we achieve true meditation, we practice it until we achieve increased unity with the eighth limb, Spirit (Samadhi). This is the highest stage of meditation. It is stated that repetition of the experience of this level culminates with total purification, perfection, and liberation.

The final stage, though not a limb, is called "Nirbikalpa Samadhi" or "Kaivala," which means, perfection, a total and permanent freedom through oneness with the Highest-Self. It is unclear how many people (if any) have reached this stage in this world, but it is believed to be an ongoing process and the ultimate evolution for all. It is a return to the truth of our being and an awaking from the illusion. Some say at this level, we choose to repeat the process all over again. Others say we may choose not to. It is also believed that one is able to assist their pupils or devotees whether in or out of the body. I will not state this as fact regardless of personal beliefs, or the reported experiences of others. This is because intellectual speculation, while admittedly can't of itself conclusively prove anything, can at least allow us to have an educated opinion. It seems that in the universe as we have defined it, where we are co-creating reality as it is experienced, this otherworldly communication may be possible in fact; or conversely, these believers may feel they are experiencing something, which is merely something they have only created. In either case, is it not beneficial? Ultimately, we are one with our source, thus the Source itself is the truest guru. Does that mean that we are our own best gurus, since we are one with the Source? Some may say not, since our ego imposter can easily lead us astray. Yet, how can we be sure we are not also being deceived by the ego of another, if we have chosen another as our guru? In any case, regardless of any deceptions, certainly we all do reach full realization of Truth ultimately. Perhaps if it truly was imperative to have a mentor or guide, we would feel drawn to one inexplicably, not against our will, of course. Or perhaps the guru is essential to some of us, but not all, depending on our own particular stage of spiritual evolution and our temperaments. The bottom line is to trust your intuition more than anything else. Let intuition (and not ego) be your guide. How can we know if we are being guided in the right direction? Do you feel an increasing sense of peace, love, joy, contentment, creativity, freedom, and unity despite circumstances? That may be a good indicator.

So now that we understand the logical process of how we experience this highest stage and discover our true and complete self, we can narrow our selection of methods down to the core essentials. Following is a review of each limb and the essence of its practice. Hopefully now you can see that complex practices are not really necessary. The ego would like you to believe that they are necessary because the more complex the methods, the more difficult it will be for you to understand and master them, thus the more time it will have to exist and control you. On the following page you will find that I have taken the eight stages or "limbs" found in the first column, then "translated" these Sanskrit names to our (simplified) English equivalent, in "layman's terms," followed in the last column by what I consider the core of the practice as it relates to our purposes. For example, looking at the Core Essence chart, you can see that "Yama" refers to the things we are supposed to avoid. That is why we would say these are the things we don't do, hence the term, "Don'ts." In order not to do certain things which we may be in the habit of doing, (even though they are not conducive to living in harmony with nature or others, and subsequently counter-productive to the goal(s) of yoga and/or meditation, we would need to exercise discipline (third column). You can follow this logic through the rest of the chart to get the idea. Hopefully this is an easy reference tool to break down seemingly abstract concepts and processes into a succinct and logical progression.

THE CORE ESSENCE OF YOGA

Limb of Yoga	*Translation*	Core Essence*
Yama	*"Don'ts"*	Discipline
Niyama	*"Do's"*	Aware action
Asana	*Posture(s)*	Hatha or exercise
Pranayama	*Breath Control*	Rhythmic breathing
Pratyahara	*Detachment*	Inversion of senses
Dharana	*Concentration*	Calm/focused attention
Dhyana	*Meditation*	Unification with object
Samadhi	*Unification*	Unified with "God"

*Specific and effective actual techniques for each of the above are listed under Chapter 8, Practical Practice.

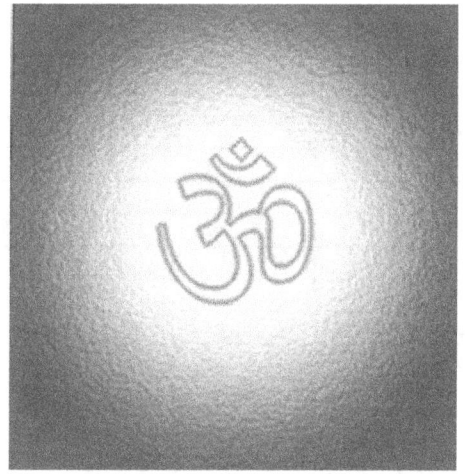

Om is composed of three semi-circles, an arc, and a dot. The first two semi-circles represent the reality you are aware of now as you read this, and the dream state. The single loop on the right side is the unconscious deep sleep state. The arc above these three is the ignorance that obstructs our awareness of Truth; represented by the dot (for Spirit), our true identity and ultimate realization.

Chapter 5

The process of evolution is not different from life itself, in that it also is a cycle. Just as for every death, there is rebirth; for every up, there is down. For every day, there is night, as the suns, stars, planets, and moons orbit each other in space. Scientists have a certain degree of understanding with planetary movements as we have learned in school. They are also able to predict cosmic events, not because they have some extraordinary gift, but due to extensive observation, documentation, and mathematic calculations. Consequently, most accept what they report as fact, even though the "facts" are ever evolving as new information is ascertained. We must be ever-ready to expand and re-examine what we think we know, in order to come nearer to the truth. There is much information in this world that may be largely unknown to particular parts of the world for various reasons, but this does not make it any less true. Just as there exist certain proven herbal or homeopathic remedies for illnesses that are not acknowledged in the United States, and other places, due to the lucrative industry of disease management, healthcare, and pharmaceuticals. (Why cure an illness, when you can get rich from sickness?) The same holds true for science and spirituality. Why educate the masses, when you can have power over them by keeping them ignorant? However, the world is still free enough to exchange information and fortunately people can still examine the evidence for themselves to decide what is, or is not true. In India and some other parts of the world, the cyclic nature of the cosmos and its relation to time and our evolution has been examined for generations. In the west, we have merely heard about astrology, which is usually quickly dismissed, thanks to the charlatans of the field, and bogus palm readers and persons with no understanding trying to make a fast profit. The reason this information is being presented at all, is for those with the curious intellect who like to learn alternative ideas in how things may work. For example: Isn't it good to know the average life expectancy of certain creatures, including ourselves? For our society, time seems so important we have put a clock in virtually every technological gadget we create. It thus seems logical to conclude that it would also be useful to know the life span of the world, of the solar system, the galaxy, even the universe, if possible. It would be good to know how it relates to our own evolution. The more we can understand the relativity of the cosmic workings around us, the easier we can become empowered and govern our lives accordingly, in harmony with the greater body. Let us now review the information and decide for ourselves.

The nearer something is to a concentration of energy, the greater the effect; just as cell phones have better signal reception in certain areas. Everything we know in this world consists of energy, as we have discussed previously. It is believed that there is a tremendous concentration of energy at the center of the galaxy. The ancient yogis have told us that our solar system travels an elliptical orbit that brings this planet in various positions of proximity to the center of the galaxy. The nearer we are to this center, the higher the level of energy we are exposed to. This affects the nervous systems of all creatures in the world. As the orbit moves away from the center, the energy diminishes gradually and corresponds to the lowest point of evolution for various species.

It is said that there are two main stellar cycles, which affect our distance from the center of the galaxy. These are the "Galactic Cycle" and "Equinoctial Cycle." Equinoctials occur in 24,000 year cycles: 12,000 "ascending," and 12,000 "descending." Galacticals occur in cycles as large as hundreds of thousands of years, but have less of a direct effect on us due to being such a long and gradual revolution. Basically, the Galactic cycle is a large orbit which carries the smaller Equinoctial orbit. Our sun with planets and moons revolves around another star in the galaxy called a "dual." As stated, this takes a total of 24,000 years to complete the orbit and simultaneously causes the backward movement of equinoctial points of the zodiac. This is what causes the variance in distance to the center. As we reach the nearest point, the center of energy, humans supposedly reach the pinnacle of evolution. After a period of being at this center, we move away from it and therefore devolve until we reach the furthest and lowest state of consciousness. This concept appears to correlate to our commonly accepted human history. If you study the Great Pyramid of Egypt beyond the watered down version presented in schools, you will find that it was built so mathematically and archaeologically exact, that the implications are astounding beyond the scope of this book. This particular pyramid was not merely a tomb. Did you know our entire mathematic system is based on it? Or, that it is aligned to the planet's grid precisely, or that it was built in direct scale and proportion to the Earth based on the formula *pi*? This occurred at a time when there were no advanced measurement mechanisms like we have today, and no way to fly either. Top scientists and engineers have concurred, that even today with all our so-called advancements, we cannot even recreate it, never mind surpass it. In fact it is even purported to have been a sort of power generator and paranormal activity facilitating mechanism. Research suggests that even if these claims are unsubstantiated, one must conclude one of two extraordinary assumptions: Either, beings of another world are responsible for its construction, or what we are discussing here is true and that we created it ourselves at our highest point of evolution. If that is true then it is implied that we are not currently at a very high stage of evolution despite what we may have thought. (Perhaps you will explore this in the future, but don't get too caught up in detail; it may distract you from the more relevant personal evolution of the self.) Our darkest time seems to be around 2,000 years ago, or around the time of Jesus. (It does not matter what your beliefs are in this matter regarding this, it is a fact that the entire world follows a calendar directly or indirectly based on the life and death of this individual.)

Each 12,000 year half of the cycle is subdivided into four "Ages." From lowest to highest age, these are as follows: In the Pre-Christian, Northern European tradition, this is known as "The Wolf, Wind, Sword, and Axe" Ages. This is like the Greek "Iron, Bronze, Silver, and Golden" Ages. For the Indo-Aryan it is known as the "Kali, Dwapara, Treta, and Satya Yugas" (Ages). The first (lowest) age lasts 1,200 years, the next, 2,400, then 3,600, finally 4,800 years for Satya Yuga. The darkest age of 1,200 years when we are farthest from the galactic energy center, we are primitive and violent people, not much more advanced than animals. In the next higher age of 2,400 years, we begin to develop an understanding of basic energy such as electricity. We begin to advance technologically. It is characterized as a materialistic time but also a transition into the next more mentally and spiritually progressive age. Does this sound familiar? This is the Age we are supposed to be in now called the "Ascending Dwapara Yuga," Ascending because we have already passed through the farthest point of the revolution and have begun to move toward the center, rather than away from it.

Think of a circle and consider the top part of it, the nearest point and our highest level of evolution. Then mark the bottom of the circle with a point to represent the farthest point and lowest evolution. Now label each side of this circle as being duration of 12,000 years.

Divide each side of the circle into 4 portions. Label each portion with the corresponding age. The top-right portion would be Satya, then below, Treta, followed by Dwapara, then finally Kali (the darkest). The top-left side will mirror the other side exactly. Keep in mind each portion will vary in size, related to its variance in duration. Such as, Satya should be the largest or longest portion. Now label each age with its corresponding duration 4,800 years for Satya. (Writing this down will aid you in understanding this concept.) Now place a small arrow on the bottom-left portion of the circle in the segment marked Ascending Dwapara Yuga, about 1/3rd of the way up. (That is where in this cycle we are supposed to be in now.) Don't worry, it doesn't necessarily mean you as an individual are limited to this particular Age. We can always transcend it if we choose. This book has this information because it is in part, meant to be a kind of handbook on life, a universal guide, or manual. Rather than be born to a world that manipulates you to become how it wants; uses and loses you in a chaotic system of power, greed, control and fear. It would be nice if one could come with an owner's manual at birth. This life-guide would say, "Here is what has been observed and believed things work, and why it is thought to be so. Have fun, choose whatever you wish; be free and fearless because there is no failure, and there is no true death. We are eternal, we may do as we please, and there are no judgments or guilt. However, there are consequences. Since we are all from the same source, everything we do eventually affects each other, one way or another."

Evolution

The next Age we are approaching is characterized by substantial maturity in mental capacity and ability: minimal ego, living in harmony with nature and communicating telepathically. This may even be possible in meditation. "How is it possible," you ask? I will tell you; regardless of whether or not I can do this, it can be logically inferred as a possibility. If you are able to sit still long enough and concentrate hard enough until your thoughts subside, your mind becomes clear, completely still and empty of thought. In this clarity, it is naturally easy to hear the mental noise of everyone else. Doesn't that make sense? But how many people actually have the discipline to practice this deeply enough? How many even if they have the ability, would be believed that they have it? If they were believed, how long would a society tolerate it before they eliminated the capable ones because they are threatened by their powers and abilities? Then again, as ever-increasing numbers of those with this aptitude procreate, the new abilities, such as mind reading, or telepathy, eventually could conceivably become part of our genetics as we evolve anyway.

In the highest age of Satya Yuga, most recently approximately in 11,500 B.C., it is believed that amazing structures (like the Great Pyramid) were created, and the spiritual science of yoga was developed as a way to maintain our ability to personally advance, despite the current age one is subjected to (as the world devolves) and still evolve individually. According to these beliefs, we have since moved away from the center for thousands of years, and have now been returning for a couple thousand years, making many technological advances. We are supposedly now about 300 years or so into the Ascending Dwapara Yuga, characterized by evolution in the fields of electronics and mechanics. This would explain the relatively recent (historically speaking), rapid advances in technology.

If we are to speculate on the purpose of a system where worlds evolve upward and downward, we can surmise that the reason would be to enable beings to experience all levels of what we are not, in order to appreciate what we are. As many of us reach the highest state, there are always others just beginning the journey. Obviously, they cannot begin that journey in a spiritually enlightened world. So then, we may also wonder, "If this cycle perpetually goes up and down, should we even bother to try to make peace in the world?" Being good is our true nature, as we evolve, it is what we choose to express. Since we are advanced, we act without attachment to results and accordingly, we do not act implicitly to save the world. Simply being peace has its own reward. Nevertheless, bringing peace and love to others is a natural and beneficial process and certainly aids the world to be less of a hellish existence for others whom are a part of you. If we did not do so, perhaps the world would not even alternate between good and bad cycles, but simply remain in a state of darkness completely. That is why it is so important for us to do our part in bringing light into this world.

Chapter 6

This chapter is intended to serve as a concise summation of the psychology of those who implement the concepts presented in these pages. The following will have more meaning if you have read up to this point and not skipped ahead. For best results, please pause to reflect on each passage.

In order to discriminate the truth from the untrue, remember that the highest thoughts, words, and feelings are those of Spirit. Anything less is from another source such as the ego. The highest thought is joy, the highest words are those of Truth, and the greatest feelings are those of love. If you seek love outside of yourself, you can be sure that you hold anger within and are afraid of it. Yet true, lasting peace will never come from the illusion of love outside of you, but only from the eternal Reality within.

The Source will send messages to us in many ways, until they are received. We will know they are from Spirit because we have never thought so clearly. If we had already thought so clearly on these questions previously, we would not be asking them to begin with.

If we can simply let go of who we are not, we shall allow ourselves to remember and embrace who we are. We can't learn that which we say we already know.

We are one all-knowing entity that has seemingly separated itself in an illusion. There is nothing to actually "learn," but only remember. We feel separate, so when we remember the truth of our nature we essentially become "one" experientially rather than conceptually, with all members and thus literally re-member. Becoming one again, we will have won.

We should see all others as an extension of the Self; however, betrayal of yourself in order not to betray another is still a betrayal. Although selflessness is the way of Spirit, it is impossible to not be selfish because all others are a part of you, and all good (or bad) comes back to you. Therefore act without attachment to results.

There is no "Law" or "Commandments" of Spirit. There are however, laws of the universe in the dynamics in how energy operates. Ergo, there are guidelines or suggestions on how we may have a better life by living in tune with these dynamics. That is balance and harmony. We were previously unaware that by transgressing these, we were inadvertently causing our own suffering. By following these guidelines we thus become freed from suffering. They are our guides to freedom, not restrictions of it.

We should try to see more in a person then what they show us. Only their fear stops them from showing us. Let them feel safe to show us what we would be wise to remember is already there. We can remind people who they are but they probably won't believe, or we can show people who they are by remembering who we are.

A great teacher is one who causes the most students to become teachers; a master is one who causes the most yogis to become masters; "God" is one whom causes all people to eventually realize they are themselves gods and also parts of one God.

All perceived problems are actually opportunities in disguise. Every moment is a gift sent from your higher-self to create yourself and your life right now. Who do we choose to be in this moment, the victim or the hero? Winning or losing isn't the point of life, loving or not is the only choice for every situation. Before you act, consider what choice will produce desired results.

Others' present faults are our own past errors, condemn no one, see the future realization in all, and by doing so, you will lead them there. Spirit wants what we want for us because it experiences itself through us. Realize this revelation now, forgive all and judge not. A system has been designed for us to experience becoming aware of who we truly are. The only difference between us and Spirit is that Spirit already knows this. We can be, do and have virtually anything we can imagine, and we attract what we fear. Like energy attracts like energy. What we resist continues to exist, but when we face our fears they disappear.

Nothing real can be destroyed, and nothing unreal truly exists. This awareness is Realization.

Fear not, failure is an illusion, because there is nothing we have to do, except remember who we truly are. Experiencing Spirit is not an unattainable goal, becoming fully aware of our eternal unity with Spirit is an unavoidable occurrence.

It may seem that we do not always get what we want, but that is because we always get what we create. If we do not like it, we can change it. We can choose again. Life is a result of our thoughts about it, including our own creative thought that we usually don't get what we want. Life proceeds from our intentions for it. We should not let shame, unworthiness, guilt or fear limit our ability to create what we want. Honor those negative feelings and then let them go. We may not understand why a door seems to be closed until the right one for our highest good opens; and therefore, we can choose and not expect, but enjoy every moment.

What does it mean, "It may seem that we do not always get what we want, but that is because we always get what we create?" Thoughts are creative and the universe is like an infinite mirror, which reflects back to us our thoughts about ourselves. The thought of wanting a thing is a statement to the universe that we do not currently have it; consequently that becomes our experience, the wanting. Instead, it is wise to be grateful, knowing all time is one and that we will have it in linear time eventually with continued, consistent, detached effort. Thankfulness is a powerful statement to Spirit. You essentially acknowledge it is ultimately already there. "Even before you ask, I shall answer." You can't fool or manipulate anyone because what you know becomes your reality. Faith is the key. The secret is to appreciate as though you already have what you would want, then the universe will respond by creating the experience of you having it already. This is why it is said that, "you can only experience what you know." If you believe in a reality in which you have no control, then that will be your experience; actually, it has been your experience, which proves that we do create our reality. Now that we know this, we can choose to experience a reality we do control.

Although the enlightened ones may choose love, it doesn't mean that they do not have other less noble attributes. Being the All, we have all qualities good and bad in order to have a full, complete experience of ourselves. Emotion is energy-in-motion. Being energy, we have e-motion. Being wise, we choose what we experience, including emotion. If we wish to experience the emotion of love, we choose to be love. We think, speak and do with love. Therefore, love becomes our experience. The question is, "What do you choose?" masters are those who consistently choose love not fear, in every moment and circumstance. Although we are in the process of experiencing our creations, we may also create the experience of not needing to experience further our creations directly, or we may choose to create from a higher consciousness. Spirit needs nothing. Since we are one with Spirit, we also should need nothing, but enjoy everything. That is freedom, accept the present and change the future.

We are already perfect, most of us are just are not remembering that and therefore not creating it, nor experiencing it yet. When we know it, we will create it and that will become our experience. That is how we define Reality. Our own minds obscure the universal truth of who we are and the ways in which our ideas are manifested. Most have not been taught that we are not the mind, but greater. We have not realized that we can operate from the higher consciousness of Spirit and thus control our minds. Remembering how to control the mind, we can consciously create our experience, rather than experience a false reality of being subjected to seemingly chaotic conditions without reason. Time is one of our creations. Why do we have birthdays and anniversaries? Can a year really repeat? What is the significance of a mass in space completing an orbit around another mass? Time is relative. There is the past, present and future. Does anything which is not now, actually occur? The circumstances of our life situation now are a result of actions of the past. Our conditions in the future will be the result of our actions in the present. Therefore, now is the only meaningful moment. There is nothing in the now that can make you feel other than you choose to feel once you realize you are able to choose what you feel, rather than be victimized by emotions. However, it is one thing to realize this conceptually, and another to master the practice of it. Yet failure is still an illusion because ultimately we are here to create without judgment, and there is no way not to create. Therefore, we are already a success. If we do not enjoy our experience we can accept the relative reality of it and re-create a new experience. Awareness, honesty, and responsibility; no limit on how great the experience can become. We create on more than one level: Physical, mental, emotional, intellectual, and spiritual. Complete mastery of life requires balance. This ensures the same thing is being created on all levels and there is no contradiction or scattered energy. Inharmonious and non-conducive habits have been formed due to much time lived in ignorance. Because of this, balance is preceded by discipline. A major part of discipline is detachment, and this means letting go of what you thought you knew, and cease telling Spirit what you think you know, so that you can receive what Spirit already knows. Then you will know because the highest part of you is Spirit. It is wise to cultivate the skill of concentration to harness your energy and efficiently focus it on creating exactly as you choose. Being your highest-self, means being love; therefore your creations will be for the highest good of all, they will be based on love. When this concentration is focused on the Self (Spirit) instead of outer creations, one becomes elevated to the highest consciousness and hence unified experientially with all that is. You experience yourself as being one with Spirit. Persistent thoughts create our reality. If we want to control it, we must control our thoughts. This is our responsibility.

Spirit is the process of love expressed through energy as a system in which we are able to create what we wish and experience our creations. Spirit *is* Life.

What does Spirit want from us? Spirit wants for us what we want for us. The absolute form of what we call Spirit seems to be love, therefore love is the only factor that is real (by definition) because Spirit's love is said to be a constant variable, unaffected by condition and thus unconditional. Human love is a mere fraction of that love and diluted by conditions and fear. Consequently, it is transitory and ultimately unreal. That is why it does not fully satisfy. Nevertheless, there must be a core of true love within us. That is also Life/Spirit. If we go within, perhaps we can locate this source of life and love. If we could find it and remain in that state, we might no longer be overly concerned with the events of this world. That is freedom. Being that freedom, we could cause others who are ready, to realize their own nature and also become free.

Spirit is whispering to us, but our minds are too loud with thought to hear it. If we can still the body and quiet the mind, we just may finally hear the universe. One of the methods we may use to achieve this stillness is Yoga Meditation. With this, the body exerts the energy it has absorbed so that more can flow through it freely. Then the physical and astral bodies become balanced and still. With control of the breath, they further become disciplined and the mind becomes quiet and serene. The senses revert to flow inwardly, rather than to the outer world and focus on the subtle currents of energy. With concentration, a deeper focus on one aspect of that energy raises the consciousness. One may actually perceive this energy, which has been referred to as "Om" or the "inner-voice." One finds that energy does not end with their body, but extends out into everything. Through detachment and concentration, we can re-associate our body-identified awareness to this energy, and our sense of self can expand. We then may experience higher levels of the self until culmination in ultimate unity with the highest-self. At that level we should realize we need nothing because we are everything by being one with it. We see with the eyes of Spirit. In this state we can infer thinking no longer becomes necessary as we have become the source of all wisdom itself. Thinking is only the mind attempting to gain information, yet becomes unnecessary when we actually become that information. This is the highest stage of meditation. The definition of yoga is, "to unite." To unite the lower, limited portion of the self to the higher, infinite existence and become whole. This is the meaning of the word, "Holy." We are the "Holy Ghosts," are we not? But to appreciate our experience, there needs to be relativity. The dualistic world provides that. There may always be those unready to become whole, but we should not judge them. They are our own past life, and we should love life. We understand the process. The cycle of life is the music of creation with its infinite levels or rhythms. In that elevated state of being, this may become your perception. But unless you remain in that state permanently, you may return here. You might have realized that the world is unreal by definition because it is changing, and only the unchangeable is true reality. Or, you may say nothing is unchangeable, so therefore everything is real since otherwise nothing would be, but that may be an unacceptable answer. You may also conclude that everything is real, but what a person perceives at any given point in their development of becoming whole, is only a small portion of the whole. This Reality is vibrating and pulsating in unimaginably creative magnitude. We created it and then submerged ourselves into the creation, forgetting what we have done.

Imagine being awake and thinking about something, only to fall asleep and dream about it, forgetting whom you are and what you have done to inspire the dream. But then you wake up and have a good laugh. You look around and there are others sleeping. They are not ready to awaken, so you let them sleep, kindly watching over them. Then there are others who are suffering from a nightmare. You gently wake them and they are grateful. You did not impose your will, because you felt their unspoken desire to be awoken. You remember your dreams but appreciate being awake. Then the awoken ones realize they have not truly awoken, but only risen to another dream level. Suddenly, you truly awaken and realize that it was only you dreaming that you were many others. The "music's over," so what else is there to do? Start the music over again. You fall asleep, again becoming confused in your dream, which you forgot you are creating. You have many questions and call out for help once again, when ironically, not only are you the question, calling to Spirit to answer you, but since you are a part of Spirit, you are your own answer.

Let's pause to meditate on this concept now.

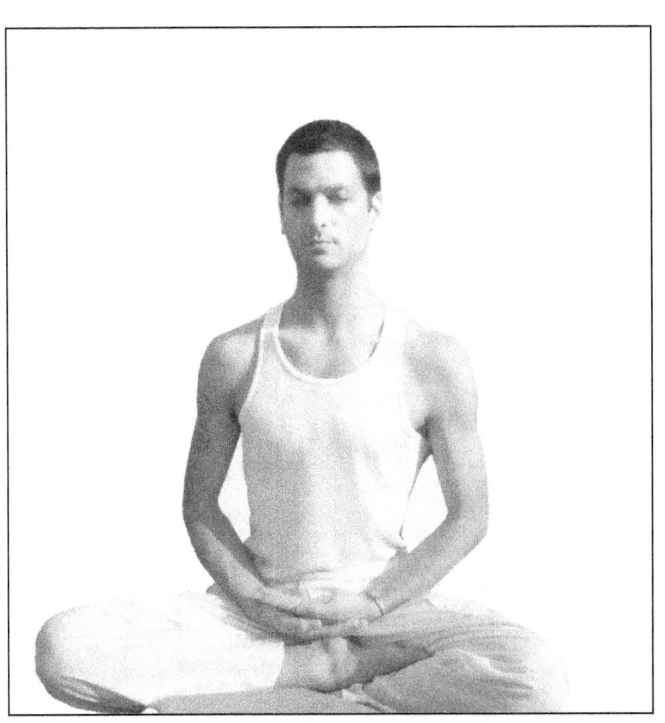

Chapter 7

-Inspired poetic work-

How can I exist in a world of shame? Once I knew no better, wild, untamed. Then somehow I came to know things with out names; the world betrays itself, cause and effect multiply; yet somehow I transformed and suddenly crossed the line- I awakened. Life is like a cycle of infinite chain reactions, each caused and affected by another with ignorant conditions. Every creature suffers sickness, age and death; and the cycle goes on and on, but why, no one can guess. We try to hide the truth with foolish work and play; we please ourselves by buying things, when in ground we shall lay. It occurred to me, you see: that everyday is the same, and the time passes endlessly until the meaning is read. We have the power to change it all, end the pain, escape; with every action, word or thought, purify the mental state. Each of us creates the world, each cause pleasure or pain. It's time to be responsible, transform the world of shame. Can't you see that all along, we were the ones to blame? So join me now my friends and don't wait another day, we've waited long enough I'd say, it's time now to awake.

* * *

They are like illusions hunting empty images, causing pain to themselves and others- raising young ones in the same. Empty creatures of flesh attack each other; ghastly ghouls seek pleasure in absurd ways. When actions carried out from fancies of mind, create the world of objects which we see around, immortals declare, "How can these humans do such wrong, yet wonder why the world's not right?" It seems obvious to me that changing minds are the solution, to ending contaminated actions, which cause this pollution. How can you exist and not question why? I know the answer's there but you don't even try. You're afraid of what you'll find out if you do; it might mean changing everything that you thought, that you knew. It's not easy to understand, but there is a reason and a plan. The purpose of life is to love the most you can, expanding yourself endlessly with your infinitely helping hands. There is no escaping yourself, so forget hiding from truth through wealth. When you pass on, it will remain here for another, you'll be born again; another time, another place, to another mother. Why waste time with impermanent satisfaction? Cleanse the mind now and observe the reaction. Recognize responsibility of positive and negative distinctions. I urge you to awaken now before we face extinction. I've seen things I can't explain. I evaporated and became the rain. I fell to this Earth and became a seed; I blossomed into a sturdy tree. I fed my friends with my fruit and leaves, but humans came and took an axe to me. They built me into a house in a cozy town; then after some time I burned to the ground. My ashes flew up into the sky; I laughed, I cried- but I never died.

* * *

Energy- the guiding force, forces humanity not aware. Always existed, always did, and by a different name always there.

God- some call it that, but why must we personify? So understand and love as much as we can before we die.

Death- when we're done, we're not through because our life after death was before, we didn't know, but now we do, new knowledge gained, forever lords.

* * *

Knowing that you're not from this world is freedom, but wisdom is acting like it. Freedom is also remembering that pain is not your name. Wisdom is playing the game; we're all the same. Everyone is trying to be so cool. Impressing each other with lies, it's the rule. All of them trying so hard to be cool; I look around and laugh because at one time I did it too. I'd like to tell you that I feel much lighter here; I've left it all behind, a liberated and unattached seer. I observe this body passing through false senses of security. It's all changes like fluid colors in the winds of my maturity. It blows through your hair and you get scared, you feel like a fool, but try to play it cool. It's the rule. Everyone is trying so very hard to be cool; trying so hard we failed to notice that we choose to lose.

* * *

I'm standing here exposed for you all to see, it took a lot of courage facing fear, now I'm free. Make your judgment, compare and criticize, "He can't dance, he can't sing, he can't fight." Blood, sweat and tears hit the floor, now I'm clean, but can you see me? I'm not what you see, your not who you think, so what is real now? If you are what you think, then tell me where do thoughts come from? If you don't know, then you also are not known. Now you see that you are not your thoughts, who you are is greater than the sum of your parts. Knowing not the originator of thought, admitting you are that which you know naught. This of all is most hard, but if you understand this you have come quite far. So stop thinking and just be, try to channel the truth and then you'll see, answering the cosmic riddle of: "Who are we?" It's the only way that we are freed.

* * *

It's a mean world; cold, critical eyes will stare and dare you to fail. Courage shall rise with intent to remind that it is everything and therefore, is you. Being one with the unseen you cannot fail, but only create, and so we must step into the spotlight, there is no other moment. It feels better to love than fear. I too was once cold, but now I won't fault them, as they are my own past Age. Now without hesitation, I shall take the stage.

* * *

The <u>Rhymes</u> of Reality

We are sleeping gods. We are gods within our own dream. We are safe within the dream; perfect in every way. The dream experiences are reflections of the individual's thoughts about itself. Until the entity remembers the truth, the law of (karmic) cause and effect continue until finished. One dreams through many, but it is not chaos. There is science in this sphere as observed in nature. You discover the science of yourself, the true self, self-realization, and real-I-zation. Self-Realization thus evolved and hastened through yoga is the art of reunion of Soul with Omni-Spirit.

* * *

Name the desire and will it to be so, remain unattached to the result. Give the power to fulfill to the mercy of another. Do not feel shame; your surrender provides them the gift of the opportunity to experience compassion. If the result doesn't turn out as you wished, thank them internally for teaching/reminding you of detachment. Be glad that you faced fear and did all that you could to create your situation and know that the decision was for the highest good of all seen and unseen in ways you may not understand. Know that regardless of outcome, you are loved and never alone as we are all one. If your wish was fulfilled, be grateful but be unattached, as easy as things come, remember things go.

* * *

How can we recognize each other, we don't remember who *we* are? *Communication.*

What is the purpose of communication? *Connection* to others.

Why do we try to connect to others? To acquire or distribute *information.*

What is the value of information? *Knowledge.*

What are we trying to know or acquire? *Ourselves,* knowledge of true selves.

Why do we try to know or acquire ourselves through *others?* ....*Ignorance.*

* * *

We love to be afraid and we're afraid to love. If Spirit is love, then we are afraid of Spirit. What we deny exists, cannot be fixed, face the fear and it disappears. Love is freedom, this is truth, and a life of living love reveals joy as proof.

Chapter 8

Based upon the tenets of the eight limbs of yoga and the simplified principals, outlined here chronologically, are detailed instructions with specific techniques for practice of yoga, followed by meditation.

Yama and Niyama

- Daily discipline of moderation in sense fulfillment such as food, drink, and entertainment. Naturally, this also includes avoiding violence, aggressive speech, thoughts and actions, moderation in sexual activity and no recreational drug use. Also, try to use all-natural and/or organic products, especially produce if locally available and feasible.

- Adhering mostly to a vegetarian diet, meaning limiting consumption of meat, eggs and some dairy by reflecting on its impure quality (toxins are released and stored in the body as it is digested) and inhumane method of acquisition, in addition to the effect on the global ecology. If you do have some meat, ensure it was not processed with rBHT, MSG, steroids, or hormones. It is also recommended to avoid chemicals & processed food items, and consider other important nutritional needs as well.

- Receive some sunlight on a regular basis, perhaps several times a week or at least a minimum of 10 minutes per day if possible, but not to be over exposed (or under-protected) to it either. Avoid the health risks associated with radiation from over-exposure.

- Daily conscious breathing, meaning full yogic breaths, (in fresh air whenever possible). This is a full and calm regulated breath that keeps you aware, detached and peaceful throughout your day. This also makes meditation easier as your body is already acclimated and the mind is serene.

- Engage in work and activity, which has a positive nature. This means thinking, speaking and doing good to others in contact with you, and making your life-work something beneficial to society, and preferably both enjoyable and lucrative. (*Money/success used properly is not bad.*)

Meditation comes naturally after one is able to successfully concentrate deeply. But deep concentration comes easier if it is preceded by physical exercise and breath control. The reasons for this were explained earlier. (Please remember that this chapter is an outlined summary of the process with the associated actual techniques. If you do not remember the reasons, please refer to the appropriate section of this book to refresh.)

Depending on your schedule, you can begin with a form of exercise. For example, if you need to spend time with your partner or family, but then will not have time for the Hatha Yoga postures later; you may wish to substitute with perhaps a couple games of tennis. This way you burn off excess toxins and allow the energy to flow through you rather than stagnate. If you don't exercise enough, your body will resist the stillness of practice later because it will either have too much stored energy or feel depleted. It could feel depleted because if you do not engage in activity, you do not use energy. If you do not use it, your body does not need to gather more from the universe as it does when you sleep. (How else do you think we recharge at night?) That is why we must be active in order to have the right balance of energy even though it may seem contradictory at first. I suggested tennis because this sport requires movement yet is not violent in nature as some other sports.

On the days that it is not possible to play a sport or go jogging, or to change the routine, you can practice Hatha Yoga postures. See the bibliography on further study of this specific area of yoga and remember that this is a step in the process, a means to an end, and not a complete practice in of itself any more than washing the dishes with complete detachment and being fully present in the moment. Meaning, practicing the positions and being fully aware are a form of meditation, but not actual meditation either because it seems unlikely that you would experience a state of total God-Realization doing that alone. I suppose it could happen (for those whose life plan allows it), but then again this book is written for the average person, not the exception.

Modern society does not have much free time and therefore usually cannot explore all the hundreds of posture variations. Time would be more efficiently spent on the complete balanced approach consisting of Hatha as a small portion thereof. It is meant as a healthy activity and preparation for meditation. Hatha is to be followed by Pranayama breathing which controls both mind and energy. It is the most important step and we will come to that shortly. When time (or physical limitations) prevent either exercise or Hatha Yoga, before meditation practice (including Pranayama), we can practice the Energization Exercises (not included here, see recommended resources). This is a 15 minute routine, which incorporates the principals of yoga. As mentioned, it was created by a well-known and (allegedly) enlightened yogi by the name of Paramhansa Yogananda, and can be learned through the Self-Realization Fellowship or other establishments such as Ananda. (Be advised that I caution against commitment to any organization above and beyond learning to some degree.) After some physical exertion, one moves on to the other limbs. Ideally one should begin with Hatha Yoga, but if not enough time, then substituted with Energization, or at least some kind of sport or exercise.

Hatha Yoga
The Sun Salutation

Go through the 12 postures, 12 times as shown on pages 144-145. This can take 15-30 minutes (or more if desired) depending on the speed at which they are performed. They should be done with an attention to the body and awareness of breath. The breath should be maintained at an even rhythm. The postures will be woven around the breath, as an excellent preliminary to Pranayama. These postures elongate the spine, rejuvenate the nerves, massage the organs, activate the glands, and are supposed to balance the chakras. They also increase flexibility and promote peace. The interesting thing is that through this discipline, one is able to relax and re-energize simultaneously. This makes for a perfect preparation for meditation. The control of the body and breath leads to control of the mind. Once this is done, we can transcend it. The following are just a few postures, but they are a complete flowing series often performed prior to doing other positions, (such as page 142), which are not shown in this text. If the reader is interested, they are encouraged to research some of the many other avenues available to learn this physical portion of yoga more deeply, (see the Bibliography); however, they are advised not to overly focus on this one branch and neglect actual meditation.

As with any exercise or diet, for your own health and safety it is recommended that you consult your physician before attempting certain methods in this book.

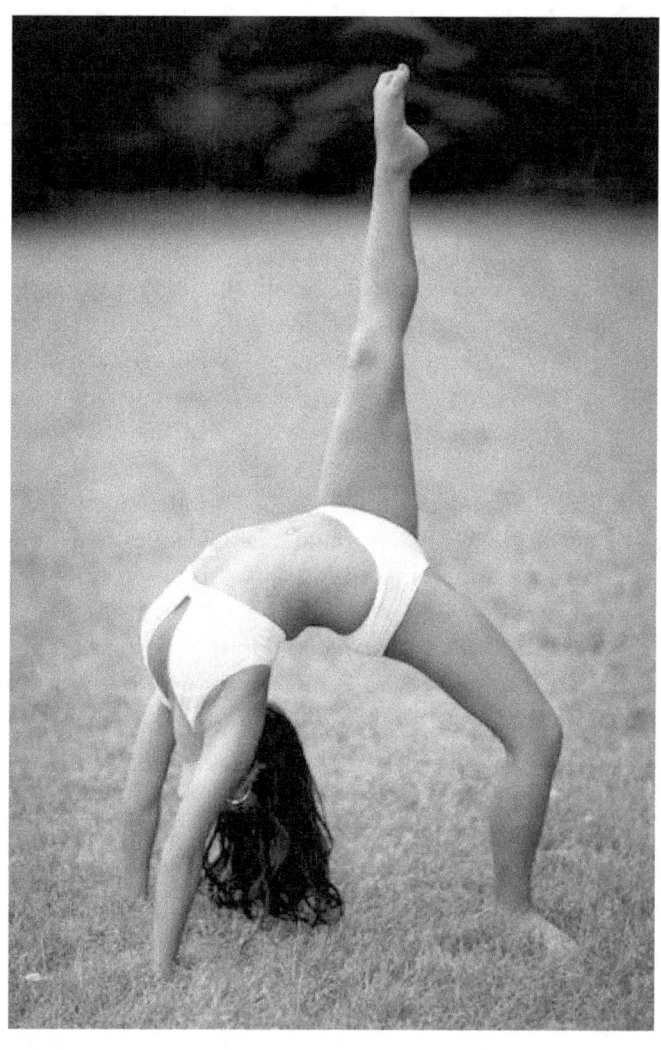

Shown above, a variation of
"Urdhvadhanurasana," (Upward Bow.)

* * *

Do not force yourself uncomfortably into positions, and do not strain yourself. Gently extend, stretch, and relax into the postures. You may wish to purchase a "Tapas" or "Sticky" Mat, for yoga practice. These are thin (1/8th inch - ¼ inch), rubbery, textured, rectangular mats used to practice Hatha Yoga postures. You can get one for $20 to $30 (at the time this is printed) at nearly any yoga center, or on the Internet.

Hatha Yoga should be performed in loose, comfortable clothing, or in tight, spandex-like material, or even in the nude; and always barefoot. The yoga mat helps one to hold a grip with hands and feet without slipping, and also provides some cushioning for the body.

* * *

1. Mountain 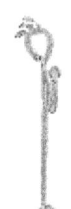 Begin by standing with feet about hip width apart, hands either by your sides or in prayer position. Take several deep breaths. Release tension, elongate spine, and come into alignment.	2. Volcano 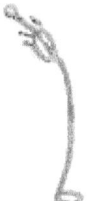 On your next inhale, in one sweeping movement, raise your arms up overhead and gently arch back as far as feels comfortable and safe.	3. Standing Forward Fold 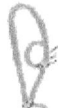 As you exhale, bend forward, bending the knees if necessary, and bring your hands to rest beside your feet. Completely relax into position and feel the body drop deeper into the fold. Let the head hang.
4. Lunge Left 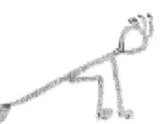 Inhale and step the right leg back, left foot forward. Feel the body stretch and foot should be between the hands.	5. Plank 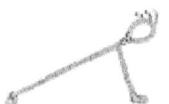 Exhale and step the left leg back into plank position. Hold the position and inhale, briefly holding the breath while in this position.	6. Stick  Exhale and lower yourself as if coming down from a pushup. Only your hands and feet should touch the floor.

7. Cobra	8. Downward Dog	9. Lunge Right
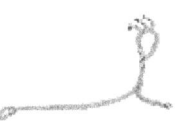	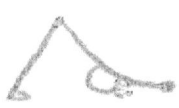	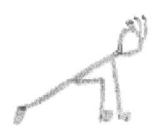
Inhale and stretch forward and up, bending at the waist. Use arms to lift the torso, bend back as far as feels comfortable. Lift legs up- only the tops of the feet and the hands touch floor. Keep arms bent, elbows pressed toward the body.	Exhale, lift from the hips and push back and up. Keep hands and feet pressed firmly into the floor. Feel the body stretch and relax. Allow the back to sink in toward the floor and the hamstrings to stretch gently.	Inhale and step the right foot forward, left leg back, feeling the body stretch. The foot should be between the hands.
10. Standing Forward Fold	11. Volcano	12. Mountain
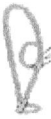	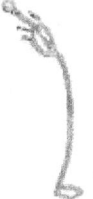	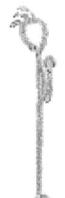
Exhale, bring the left foot forward and step into forward fold once again. Completely relax into position and feel the body drop deeper into the fold. Let the head hang.	Inhale and rise slowly while keeping arms extended. Raise your arms up overhead and gently arch back as far as feels comfortable and safe.	Exhale, and in a slow, sweeping motion, lower arms to the sides. End by bringing your hands up into prayer position. Repeat sequence, stepping with other leg 1st.

Preliminary Meditation Steps:
Pranayama to Samadhi

- Avoid eating 2-3 hours before practice.
- Choose a clean/quiet place where you will not be disturbed. Preferably, face north or east, as it is believed the Earth's energy flows in these directions, making energy control easier.
- Choose a solid, stable chair of proper height in proportion to your physique, the chair neither too high nor too low. Add cushioning for adjustments and comfort if needed. If you can sit comfortably for meditation in the "lotus," "half-lotus," or cross-legged position, then do so. If not, proper posture and alignment seated in a chair or on any structure which provides adequate stability and comfort is completely acceptable. It is believed that placing a wool and/or silk blanket under your chair or self, helps to deflect the negative gravitational pull of the earth, making easier the elevation of consciousness.
- During breath control, the body will become warm, but during meditation it becomes cool. It is advised to place a thin garment such as a light rectangular drapery over the shoulders, covering the back like a shawl. This helps to contain the positive energy you will be generating and keep the body warm during the cooling effect of meditation, thus also preventing catching a cold.

Pranayama

- If possible, sit straight so that the energy can flow freely within you. Remain still. Keep the body steady, straight, aligned but relaxed.
- Close your eyes and exhale completely, pulling in your abdomen to squeeze out all the air as though you were ringing out a sponge.
- Focus your gaze gently at the sixth chakra also known as the third eye or spiritual eye. This is the point between the eyebrows and just above where the nose connects to the forehead. Your gaze should be specifically at an imaginary point an arms length in front of this area. This means the eyes will be looking upward slightly, but not crossed. Where your attention is, your energy follows, and the goal here is to bring the energy from the base of the spine to travel upward through the spine and connect to the third eye. Conversely, you may choose instead to simply close your eyes and/or focus on the heart center, or even on the energy surrounding your physical body. The goal, uniting the lower consciousness with the higher one.
- Inhale slowly through the nose, gently expanding the inner throat (the mouth is closed), deeply filling your lungs. Do not strain yourself. If done properly, you will notice a wind-like sound stream through the throat. You should feel the air against the back of the throat.

- As you inhale, count mentally until you reach the limit of lung capacity. Feel the lungs expand the abdomen, then the rib cage, and finally the chest.
- Begin to exhale slowly through the nose, and counting mentally to the same number as before. Pull in the abdomen once again to expel all the air.
- Be sure to have the count of inhalation and exhalation to be the same. You may notice a slight sensation of coolness in the throat (and eventually the spine) as you breathe in; and slight heat sensations as you breathe out. This is attributed to the ida/pingala nadis upward and downward currents of energy.
- 12 rounds or 10-15 minutes of this breath work is sufficient.

[Example: Inhale to a count of 12 and exhale to a count of 12, for 12 rounds if possible.]

It is purportedly possible to balance and control this energy with practice in order to raise the kundalini and activate the chakras. The "advanced" teachings, state that when ready, your consciousness or Spirit will perceive a golden ring of light at the point of the sixth chakra, with a dark blue/black sphere inside and a white 5 pointed star in the middle. Your consciousness will then (allegedly) travel through it, having various experiences as it temporarily leaves the body. In the advanced Kriya Yoga teachings, however, it is taught that that one should revolve the energy around the spine also, as these revolutions purify ones karma, thus hastening their evolution. But for now you only need to be concerned with these steps to the extent that they produce peace, calmness, and concentration. Love, wisdom, joy, balance, experiences, abilities, and evolution will come of their own accord. If you were to practice with the intent of having these experiences solely, they will not be had. That is because the ego is the opposite of Spirit. What I mean is, it is a tool of Spirit and therefore to follow the desires of the ego will not lead you to the realm of Spirit. Only following the ideals of the Soul, can you experience the Spirit. Therefore, do not get excited about the details and complexities too early or you risk not properly mastering each stage before proceeding to the next. I have found abstract, intellectual knowledge of Truth to be virtually useless, as it does not increase control of emotions, or increase peace, love and joy. It may actually have the reverse effect of causing one to erroneously feel superior to others and the world, or to feel that nothing really matters. This of course is untrue, so please heed this warning, which I myself wasted much time over. Keep in mind that regardless of the validity of the existence of chakras, kundalini, or even the spiritual eye, focusing on these or anything (preferably internal) can aid the meditative process. Whether chakras "activate," or kundalinis "rise" is secondary to the actual elevation and expansion of consciousness to unite with the Infinite Self.

Pratyahara

When you control the breath, and concentrate deeply, eventually the senses, which are a physical manifestation of an outward flow of energy, are reversed inwardly. When this occurs, one is no longer aware of the objects of sense. You no longer hear or notice external sounds, no longer see, or perceive anything other than the object of concentration such as the breath and maybe the sixth chakra (and/or perhaps Om). When the mind is no longer disturbed by these distractions, it is able to concentrate more deeply. This is not so much a step as it is a phase in the process. It is a result of success in controlling the breath and energy. By becoming serene and watchful in sitting practice and controlling the breath, you are able to become increasingly aware of ever-deeper levels of control. The breath becomes increasingly still until one begins to perceive more subtle currents of energy beneath the usual act of breathing. Since at some point, you have gained a mastery of breathing, once you become aware of the subtle energy currents of energy (prana), you find yourself able to control it. This occurs as you concentrate. Your attention directs the inward flow of energy. This is how the senses cease to disturb you. Once this happens it becomes easier to concentrate. As you concentrate without distractions from the senses, you are able to go deeper within more quickly. It is possible that one may progress from control of breath to concentration directly, with Pratyahara (sense withdrawal) occurring as result at some point, and followed then by an even deeper concentration; a seemingly simultaneous process. However, in actual practice, it seems less complex to me to state that one goes from Pranayama to Dharana, with Pratyahara occurring within Dharana.

Dharana

- Release control of the breath and breathe naturally. Do not control it. Continue to sit straight with the eyes closed and remain without motion.
- Simply observe the breath flowing in and out of the body. Watch it in a detached way, as though you were observing someone else breathing.
- Do not worry about time; Let go of the body. Just be, the "watcher."
- As the breath moves in, mentally sound: "Om." This is a verbal representation of energy; being the root sound of all words, it comes closest to recreating the sound of this energy. This also helps to detach from the thoughts and the mind.
- As the breath moves out, again repeat "Om." The significance of this sound has been explained previously.
- The breath is calm now and so are the thoughts, this makes concentration easier already. If one has become able to invert the senses at will, even better. If not, it will occur eventually in concentration mode. When it does, the concentration becomes deeper, and the subject

(you), object of concentration (Om, spiritual eye, etc.), and the awareness of the act of concentration become one. Your consciousness temporarily re-identifies itself with the object of concentration. When this occurs it is no longer Dharana, but has become Dhyana.

Do this for at least 10 to 15 minutes after the 12 times (or 10-15 min.) of Pranayama breathing.

Dhyana

This deepest concentration has become true meditation. The process will progress to practice repetition in reaching this stage; and the goal then becomes making the object of meditation, your highest-self. The Om technique and all previous stages or limbs help one to achieve this because they are all various levels of concentration. The process of yoga is intended to essentially prepare and condition one to sit still for sufficient time, to remain calm and unperturbed, to detach from the body and quiet the mind by turning off the senses which cause emotion and thought. One then proceeds to become aware of, and eventually control energy to further increase concentration to the point of being able to place the awareness anywhere chosen.

Samadhi

It is then realized that it is just one more step to choose the most appropriate point of conscious unification, Spirit. When this occurs, true definition of yoga is reached, union of Soul and Spirit as one, once again. This is Samadhi. This is the return to your truest self-awareness: pure existence, consciousness, and bliss. At this stage, you are said to realize your infinite love, joy, and wisdom. You no longer fear death as you have experienced it. The only death that exists is the death of a false sense of self. The new one is eternal and free. Yet, it is said that we can still live in the world and use our ego as a tool. We can live here until it is our time to go to the next world. Just reaching this level is not perfection because we may (theoretically) still be pulled back due to our unfulfilled karma. There is a cause and effect relationship that we created in our minds with all our desires and reactions, which need to be played out, unless they don't, "Divine Grace?" That is why the advanced yogis state that there are higher levels of Samadhi before we are completely and permanently freed. Also, there are the teachings mentioned previously in which one practices certain techniques of revolving the energy around the spine to accelerate this process. Kriya Yoga can be researched with caution via the Bibliography if the reader chooses. However, remember my warning, the ego loves to entertain us with desires to accomplish difficult tasks and intellectual understandings, but they are of no use to us spiritually. Ego successes die with the ego, spiritual successes stay with us from life to life. My opinion is that the "advanced" aspect of yoga, if even valid, is unnecessary for our intents. It does not matter ultimately how much you have possessed or accomplished in life, but only how much you have loved. So, love every moment, and every difficulty; never feeling guilty for your perceived shortcomings or failures. Failure is an illusion. Remember, ultimately we are already free; yoga and meditation just help us to experience it. With that perception, you can proceed to live life to the fullest, go after what you want and be successful. Just don't depend on the outer circumstances or internal reactions to determine who you are. Begin with knowing and creating, proceed to being and experiencing, and then end without ever ending. Yoga Meditation is one of the methods we can incorporate to assist us.

SUMMARY OF PRACTICE

1. **Yama**- Don'ts, <u>Discipline.</u>

2. **Niyama**- Do's, <u>Aware Action</u>.
    - Daily Moderation & Balance with Detachment.
    - Proper Breathing (full, regulated breath.)
    - Vegetarian Diet (limited meat, some dairy.)
    - Proper Exercise & no drugs, some sunlight.
    - Positive Thought, Speech, & Aware Action (with forgiveness.)

3. **Asana**- Posture, <u>Hatha postures or exercise.</u>
    - Do not eat 2 – 3 hours before practice.
    - Choose a clean and quiet place where you will not be disturbed.
    - Choose a solid, stable chair of proper height in proportion to your physique or sit in lotus, half-lotus, or cross-legged position.

4. **Pranayama**- Breath Control, <u>Rhythmic Breathing.</u>
   - If possible, sit straight so the energy can flow freely within you. Remain still.
   - Keep the body steady, straight, aligned but relaxed.
   - Close your eyes and exhale completely, pulling in your abdomen to squeeze out all the air as though you were ringing out a sponge.
   - Focus your gaze at the sixth chakra also known as the third eye or spiritual eye; or your aura, etc.
   - Inhale slowly through the nose, gently expanding the inner throat (the mouth is closed), deeply filling your lungs. Do not strain your self. If done properly, you will notice a wind-like sound stream through the throat. You should feel the air against the back of the throat.
   - As you inhale, count mentally until you reach the limit of lung capacity. Feel the lungs expand the abdomen, then the rib cage, and finally the chest.
   - Begin to exhale slowly also through the nose, and once again counting mentally to the same number. Pull in the abdomen to expel all air.
   - Be sure to have the count of inhalation and exhalation to be the same.
   - 12 rounds or 10-15 minutes of this is sufficient.

5. **Pratyahara**- Detachment.
   <u>Inversion of the senses during concentration.</u>

6. **Dharana**- Concentration.
   <u>Calm focused attention to an object or energy.</u>
   - Release control of the breath and breathe naturally. Do not control it. Continue to sit straight with the eyes closed and remain without motion.

- Simply observe the breath flowing in and out of the body. Watch it in a detached way, as though you were observing someone else breathing.
- Do not worry about time; forget about it, there is no time. There is nothing you need to do and nowhere that you must go. Let go of the body. Just be, "the watcher."
- As the breath moves in, think the word "Om," which is a verbal representation of energy. Being the root sound of all words, it comes closest to recreating the sound of this energy. This also helps to detach from the thoughts and the mind.
- As the breath moves out, again repeat "Om." The significance of this sound has already been explained.
- Do this for at least 10 to 15 minutes after the 12 times (or 10-15 min.) of Pranayama breathing.

7. **Dhyana**- Meditation.
   Unification with the object of concentration.
   - The concentration becomes even deeper, subject (you), object of concentration (Om, spiritual eye, etc.), and the awareness of the act of concentration become one. Your consciousness temporarily re-identifies itself with the object of concentration. Thus, it goes beyond concentration to true meditation.

8. **Samadhi**- Unification.
   Unified with Spirit as the object of concentration.
   - The goal then becomes making the object of meditation, God/Spirit/Your Highest-Self.

Chapter 9

At the time this book is written, the people of this world suffer from global afflictions such as, crime, violence, terrorism, starvation, poverty, disease, war, natural disasters, and many other calamities. These unfortunate events are regularly reported in the news media, but there are many positive things happening in the world too which are not nearly as thoroughly covered. Reforms, education, peace, personal success, financial prosperity, scientific discoveries, technological advances, progress in medicine, increased productivity and efficiency, increased spiritual awareness, popularity of yoga, and much more are but some examples. This impacts the world in ways most of us do not realize. Everything we are exposed to through the senses, affects us. Most of us are not aware that the media (just like religion and politics), has realized the profitability in fear. They are feeding humanity negative images and horror stories on a daily basis. In fact, I refer to the nightly news as the "Death Report." They keep us watching to see what bad things happened to others and could happen to us at any time. What they may or may not realize is that this irresponsibility is contributing to our society becoming a fearful and depressed one. We

157

no longer believe we can change the system, which we have ourselves created. We believe there is nothing we can do about big issues such as poverty and war. Could this be because it is the government that controls the media? We are programmed by it. How and why would they do this? Television personalities and staff members that do the reports work for the network which broadcast the information to you, and the programming is financed through commercials that are paid for by large corporations. Further, the network itself is owned by still larger conglomerates. Then we have politicians whom are elected by voters, right? But how do the people know who to vote for? Ironically, we usually vote based on who we know from the television commercials. Where do the politicians get the money to pay for these expensive advertisements? Money often comes from supportive corporations through campaign contributions. So, when these elected officials are writing laws for us to follow, are they making them in our interests, or for those who have paid for them to have the office which they do? Once they have this power, how can they be sure to maintain it? Power is kept by keeping society ignorant of the truth. What is the truth they want to hide from us? The truth they hide is our own individual and collective power. They also try to hide from us how to build wealth because they fear that if we had it, they no longer would. How can they attempt to keep us ignorant of the truth? Through the same media, which gave them their power to begin with, they use the news to report to us what they want. They program us with nationalism, sensationalism, consumerism, celebrity, gossip, and fear. They do not allow us to feel our godliness, our unity, and our power. They want us to feel afraid and separate. They want us to disagree, and be addicted to the senses or afflicted by emotion. They scare or distract us. Then we justify underpaying our educators and overpaying sports and entertainment figures.

The problem with the media and how it affects us is primarily the violence. It is everywhere, from TV to movies to video games, sports, and music. Must we really wonder why our kids imitate it, or adults act it out. Is it really a mystery why we see it on the street? We report on it and watch it in the news, creating an endlessly repetitious cycle. Why aren't we learning from our journalists about how to protect ourselves, how to get affordable education, how to improve and help each other? They want people to keep buying the newest and best electronics, or vehicles and to dream of being a celebrity, but struggle just to exist here. They keep the public enticed so no one will realize how far they have fallen. If fortunate, we can go to a good college but the only way to get there is to pay for it with a big loan with lots of interest. Then when we get out and finally get a job, we go to work with a car we also had to finance and pay taxes on; then we buy gas for it, which they control the price of, and we pay taxes on this as well. We get the first paycheck and then they take more money from that also. Then with what remains, we go to buy the things they programmed us to want, and they take even more with retail sales tax. We turn on the television and hear the horror of the world, feel afraid, and drug ourselves on silly sitcoms, falling asleep to do it all again the next day. We slave at jobs we mostly dislike so the wealthiest 1% can flit about the world doing as they please. They want you to believe there is no other way; or even that it is the best way. It isn't true. What if everyone suddenly realized their own immortality? What if we united and made a new collective choice? Could we choose a world where we need no rulers pretending to be leaders? Could we lead ourselves guided by love for one another? Is it too late to reform the country or the world, or will the world reform itself eventually, causing our human extinction through natural disasters and other global consequences? There is no point to have a revolution in the old sense of the word. This has usually been proven to yield another new but similar format. We must awaken ourselves and then each other. But words must be followed through with action. Meaning, we should not only talk of self-reform/transformation, we must do it. We must not merely preach, but practice. We should not only speak or write of meditation, we must practice it. We should not only speak of doing good things for others; we must do good things. We also shouldn't turn to scriptures for which we have no proof that anyone enlightened wrote them; or which can be misinterpreted or manipulated to justify un-godly acts. Look within and beyond selfish egotistical desires. Think logically what is best for all and act to achieve it by means of peace. How? Just be good to others. Educate yourself and others, live a life of helping people. Are you rich? How about dedicating money earned after a certain point towards positive development for others, helping others to achieve what you have. If you make millions or billions every year, when is it ever enough?

Let's say anything over 100 million earned in your life goes back to the world? Is that asking too much? How can anyone enjoy an extravagant lifestyle when others are suffering? The multi-millionaire and billionaires of the world that neglect others are greatly contributing to the destruction of civilization. How? By greedily hoarding, they are indirectly causing crime. The only real value to your life is the good you accomplished in the short time you are on this planet, not how good you lived. It seems logical to surmise that if you led a greedy life here, your next life will be designed to teach you this. How else can this be accomplished unless you will then live a poor life? If you expand your perspective of the true length of a life span, which we assume is beyond this life and includes all our lives, it seems such a waste to be concerned with the accumulation of material things and activities. By doing so, you are committing yourself to a lifestyle of the extreme opposite. The irony is that the individuals that have been concerned with keeping the masses in ignorance have ultimately caused their own ignorance and will probably find themselves subjected to the very life they forced upon others eventually. That is the beauty in the idea of karma. It is the only way to guarantee that eventually everyone will return to the source and act as one. Doing to others exactly as they would want done to them. Does there need to be starvation? Of course there doesn't. Couldn't a few billionaires come together, form a plan, and modernize those parts of the world that suffer the most? Couldn't they simply create agriculture, industry and education for them rather than just send some bags of rice? But do they want to? That is the real

161

question. They will tell you it is not possible; but is that what your intuition tells you? What else can we do more immediately to change the system? We can stop supporting it. Would manufacturers continue making tobacco if people stopped buying it? Of course they wouldn't. We should cease electing to power those whose main agenda is more wealth and power for themselves. We might change our lives to live in harmony and peace.

It is not intended for this chapter to sound radical, revolutionary, or unpatriotic. Maybe the powers that be are unwitting victims themselves of the real culprit that affects us all: Desire. By this, it is not being suggested that we eliminate all desire and have a non-passion for life, creativity, or action. Desire as we have defined it, means a hunger or greed from attempting to derive happiness through appeasing solely the senses, rather than from within. It is a desire born of egoic attachment. We have learned that we are the source of our happiness and we can properly enjoy the world through the senses once we have experienced the Source through a process such as Yoga Meditation. Then we can be in the world without forgetting we are from beyond it. We can be here without fear, because we can never disappear. Certainly the leaders of this world are ignorant themselves of the same Truth they are trying to keep us from, but intuitively know must exist. But perhaps they themselves are acting only out of selfish desire, oblivious to the karmic consequences of their detrimental actions on society. But are they not also essentially our own creation since we are the creators of our reality? Can we be forced to do anything we did not plan on some level to experience for reasons we may not fully comprehend? Didn't we plan to be born to a world where we knew we would suffer so that we could one day reflect on it from a state of enlightenment, fully appreciating what it means to be free? However, that does not mean we cannot change our choice. Haven't we had enough of this? Isn't it time for a change? Are we ready? Can we make a new choice for global enlightenment and freedom and take positive action with awareness and love, yet with detachment? If so, do you want to know what the most important thing you can do to improve the world is? *Improve yourself.*

Personal Finance

You are a part of this world for now. Like it or not, the system we use in this world is based on money. The amount of physical freedom we enjoy is undeniably due in part to money. Although we have discussed the great wrongs being perpetrated upon us by the greedy, there is a good side to money and nothing inherently wrong with having it. We need it to send our kids to the best schools, visit other parts of our planet and to provide the necessities and luxuries of human life. It is okay to have the fine things in life, provided we don't feel that we need them in order to be happy and as long as we avoid causing pain to others in order to have these for ourselves. One way to improve ourselves (and consequently our Reality) is to become educated in the fields of Business and Economics.

Some of the world's richest people attempt to enslave us by limiting our ability to learn about finance while also exploiting our sense fulfillment desire. They do this by making us want to live beyond our means and take on too much credit debt, thus paying interest to them. If you want to succeed on all levels of being, not only must you do all you can to remain physically healthy, and perform Yoga Meditation for your mind and Soul, but you should master business in general, and specifically, money. They are physical forms of energy too, after all. Remove negative patterns in your mind about success and instead create a positive association with it. Believe you will have what you need. Know that beyond linear time, you already have it. This will become your experience regardless of the obstacles others attempt to place on you. Opportunity will be created, but you must be prepared to accept it when it arrives. That means educating yourself in the appropriate fields of study to become qualified for the opportunity for which you seek. Do not allow yourself to have debt. Rather than pay interest to others, find ways to create that which will eventually self-generate more money for you with limited time investment. Learn how to make money rather than lose it. Find out what you need to invest in the stock market and/or other areas of business where your services or products will earn for you on an ongoing basis and accumulate, compounding interest over time. Prepare for your future now. Don't depend on anyone else to do it for you. It won't come effortlessly, so be the First Cause. We create our Reality and our opportunities, but don't forget the Truth while you do this. Enjoy the process.

The below steps, (with a meditative perspective) will help you create financial success and freedom:

- *Think* of your desire.
- *Determine* how much money you need.
- *Decide* that it must be so.
- *Believe* that it will happen.
- *Prepare*; exert effort to make it so.
- *Focus* your mind; be clear and ready.
- *Recognize* the opportunity when it comes.
- *Take* proper action at the right time.

Returning to the topic of worldly affairs, we said that by improving yourself, you have already done your part to improve the world. If you are not ready to do so, do not feel guilty; but how much suffering will you need to experience, or see others experience, before it reaches a level that you finally consider unacceptable? Our world is like our child as well as our habitat, if we lose it due to pollution or war, won't it be too late for humanity here? It may not be the eternal aspect of our being, but it certainly serves our purpose to create and experience in this world; and its value is worth preserving. It is arrogant to think that the world can handle whatever we do to it. However, the spiritually aware person may contemplate if it really matters, when we may reincarnate to this or another world anyway? Well, don't you think all worlds go through cycles of light and darkness regardless of what the inhabitants have realized? Look within for the answer. I have done so, and feel that it's all about choices. Do you choose to be a victim or a hero? Do you allow yourself to be manipulated by a greedy system and become a victim to it? Many have chosen this and are suffering because they are not aware of another option; those are the ones we try to reach and awaken. When they do, they feel a glimpse of freedom and unity and attempt to awaken others. They then have chosen to become the hero, the liberators of a world shrouded in darkness. Once you know the game, you will not live the same. It may be true that the world passes through stages. But one thing that even the scriptures have repeated to us is that we have always had "free will." Hence, it is not necessarily the stage of evolution for a planet which determines the level of spirituality of the individual. Planets such as this one are the hosts for Souls on a similar plane of conscious awareness and/or potentiality to live, become reminded of their truth, and make subsequent choices from that creative state of being. Therefore, if it were not for the people who choose to be "freedom fighters," the world might not be a cycle of light and dark, but only of dark. Therefore, rise and realize we are all from the same source, which makes us one. Let's change ourselves to think, speak and act from awareness and love; to help each other so that in this way the system is naturally changed. Do not fear the negativity seen in the world; society has been living in ignorance for so long, that a lot of damage has been done. Things may unravel and decay in order to make way for the new world which evolves to the next stage of enlightenment to reflect our improved understanding. A spiritual one which you may imagine exists for all life forms, even those on other worlds. It is not conducive to spiritual growth if the paranormal or extra-terrestrial is obsessed upon, even though these things most likely exist. I have noticed many tell untrue stories of otherworldly experience creating fear. Unfortunately, most of the persons speaking about this sort of thing have only financial motives. There are some on a spiritual path who start to become aware of the potentiality of super-natural phenomenon, only to have allowed themselves to become deceived, manipulated, or taken advantage of in any number of ways. Once they realize the deception, these seekers then lose faith in the truth. Potential cosmic abilities and experiences are not directly relevant to our spiritual growth and can even have a negative impact in some cases, just as all forms of energy can prove either beneficial or detrimental. There is no need to be concerned with outer-world realities other than to ascertain a general understanding of how it may all work and where we fit in to the scheme of things. It is fine to entertain such avenues of thought on occasion but not to over-indulge in it. Perhaps some may find scientific/historic value in discussing these things. But personally, I have found it counter-productive to spiritual growth. This is because most people feel discussion of these concepts are mere childish fantasy, and hence prove harmful to our reputation of credibility. Others still feel afraid of the possibilities, or become overly concerned with it, rather than make effort in the actual process of revealing Truth through yogic means. We have the power to triumph over any difficulty and negativity. We must remember that we truly are part of Spirit, which is with us at all times because it is what we consist of. Just because we have chosen the experience of being individuals in this life, doesn't mean we have to

167

choose to live in ignorance forever. When we realize death is nothing to fear, but still love being here now, we will have become quite evolved, and possibly near to enlightenment. Once we have the super-conscious experience such as from meditation, we no longer allow subconscious patterns or external stimuli to control us and our lives, or at least reduce their ability to. This means that we are freeing ourselves by regaining control of the mind, and then surpassing it through being knowledge, rather than chasing after it. We then know that we are the creator of, and partner with Life. This knowing empowers us to create what we want when we can, and at the very least choose how we experience it when we can't. Meditation becomes a part of our life, but then life itself becomes our meditation. You don't need to become enlightened to enjoy greater success in life; you only need to apply the concepts you read here and find a way to believe in your goals, and take proper and mindful steps to achieve them. This is the key to enjoy an empowered and *truly* successful life. So, use the information here to fully realize who you are, to choose who you want to be, and why you want to be here. In this moment, the only Reality is you, but the expanded perspective of "you" includes all others and all things. All are an extension of you at various levels of awareness and potential. The infinite power of the universal Source is pulsing through you. Life is a resource at your service. Freedom is now and your experience is your choice. There's only one last question:

What do you choose?

May we never again forget who we are and why we are here, as we flow through the process of life; these, our Rhythms of Reality.

DISCIPLINE,
DETACHMENT,
DEVOTION,
CONCENTRATION/MEDITATION,
FORGIVENESS,
AWARENESS,
PEACE, LOVE, JOY, TRUTH, WISDOM &
SUCCESS.

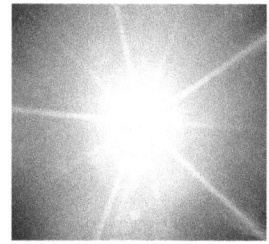

APPENDIX: Chakras
THE *EXTENDED* CHART

Please note: The chakra related information is included for interest only and has not been proven to be valid, nor important to the methods of yoga meditation presented.

CHAKRA 7: Sahasrara

Location -	Crown-brain
Color-	Violet
Gland -	Pineal
Element -	Truth/Light
Quality -	Wisdom
Planet -	Uranus
Zodiac -	Aquarius
Gem -	Amethyst/Quartz
Note -	B Note
Sense -	Beyond
Trait -	Fasting/Sun
Condition -	Wisdom
Scent -	Frankincense
Function -	God-Sat-Sat-Father Existence
State -	Spirit- The Source
Yoga Branch -	Raja/Kriya Yoga
Patanjali Yoga Applied-	Nirbikalpa Samadhi-Kavailya
Essence of Technique-	Permanent Perfection

CHAKRA 6: Ajna

Location -   Cervical-forehead
Color-   Indigo
Gland -   Pituitary
Element -   Thought
Quality -   Intuition
Planet -   Neptune/Jupiter
Zodiac -   Sagitarius/Picies
Gem -   Amethyst
Note -   A Note
Sense -   6th Sense
Trait -   Breath
Condition -   Knowledge
Scent -   Hyacinth
Function -   Cosmic Consciousness
State -   The Soul (Spirit's Reflection)
Yoga Branch -   Laya/Tantra
Patanjali Yoga Applied- Samadhi
Essence of Technique-   Self-Realization

CHAKRA 5: Visuddhi

Location -	Laryngeal-throat
Color-	Blue
Gland -	Thyroid
Element -	Ether
Quality -	Communicate
Planet -	Mercury
Zodiac -	Gemini/Virgo
Gem -	Turquoise
Note -	G Note
Sense -	Sound
Trait -	Fruit
Condition -	Harmony
Scent -	Chamomile
Function -	Soul-Om-Ananda-Holy Ghost
State -	Bliss
Yoga Branch -	Bhakti
Patanjali Yoga Applied-	Dhyana
Essence of Technique-	Meditation

CHAKRA 4: Anahata

Location -   Cardiac-chest-thoracic
Color-   Green
Gland -   Thymus
Element -   Air
Quality -   Love
Planet -   Venus
Zodiac -   Libra/Taurus
Gem -   Emerald
Note -   F Note
Sense -   Touch
Trait -   Vegetable
Condition -   Love (same as Quality)
Scent -   Rose
Function -   Intellectual
State -   The Ego
Yoga Branch -   Jnana
Patanjali Yoga Applied-   Dharana
Essence of Technique-   Concentration

CHAKRA 3: Manipura

Location -   Solar-abdomen-lumbar
Color-   Yellow
Gland -   Pancreas
Element -   Fire
Quality -   Will Power
Planet -   Mars/Sun
Zodiac -   Aries/Leo
Gem -   Yellow Citrine
Note -   E Note
Sense -   Sight
Trait -   Carbohydrates
Condition -   Will power
Scent -   Bergamot
Function -   The sense mind
State -   Sub conscious- Astral
Yoga Branch -   Mantra
Patanjali Yoga Applied- Pratyahara
Essence of Technique-   Detachment

CHAKRA 2: Svadhisthana

Location -	Sacral-pelvis
Color-	Orange
Gland -	Adrenals
Element -	Water
Quality -	Emotion/Sex
Planet -	Pluto
Zodiac -	Cancer/Scorpio
Gem -	Golden Topaz
Note -	D Note
Sense -	Taste
Trait -	Liquid
Condition -	Allegiance
Scent -	Jasmine
Function -	Vital
State -	Sub conscious- Astral Karma
Yoga Branch -	Karma
Patanjali Yoga Applied-	Pranayama-Hatha
Essence of Technique-	Proper Breath

CHAKRA 1: Muladhara

Location -	Coccygeal-base
Color-	Red
Gland -	Sex Organs
Element -	Earth
Quality -	Survival
Planet -	Saturn
Zodiac -	Capricorn
Gem -	Tigers Eye
Note -	C Note
Sense -	Smell
Trait -	Protein
Condition -	Allowance
Scent -	Myrrh
Function -	Physical
State -	Gross matter
Yoga Branch -	Conscious-Physical
Patanjali Yoga Applied-	Yama/Niyama/Hatha
Essence of Technique-	Positive Action/Exercise

RECOMMENDED RESOURCES

- **<u>Practicing the Power of Now</u>**
  Eckhart Tolle

- **<u>Conversations With God</u>** - **<u>Book 1</u>**
  Neale Donald Walshe

- **<u>The Yoga Book</u>**
  Steven Sturgess

- **<u>Autobiography of Yogi</u>**
  Paramahansa Yogananda

- **<u>The Holy Science</u>**
  Swami Sri Yukteswar

- **<u>Complete Illustrated Book of Yoga</u>**
  Swami Vishnu-Devananda

- **<u>The Yoga Sutras of Patanjali</u>**
  Translated version by Swami Satchitananda

- **<u>The Bhagavad Gita</u>**
  Translated version by Paramahansa Yogananda

- **<u>Being Nobody, Going Nowhere</u>**
  Ayya Khema

- **<u>Tao Te Ching</u>**
  Lao Tsu, translated by Stephen Mitchell

* * *

The author is not compensated in any way by these recommended resources. Some of these texts may advocate a particular religion or institution. This author is not recommending the institution or religion of their affiliation, only the general wisdom within the literature.

In addition, there are also many books and videos to be found in the general marketplace: in stores, yoga centers, and the Internet. Readers are encouraged to find and use natural products for a balanced, healthy, organic, and mainly vegetarian lifestyle.

Please do not substitute the advice in this book for professional medical counsel, treatment or procedures.

* * *

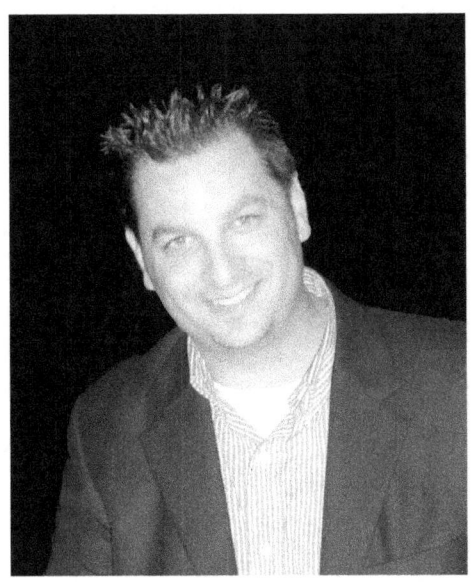

A Word from the Author

Steve hopes readers will find this book a valuable resource for discovering the key to health, happiness and success which he has attributed in part to the philosophy and methods presented in this book. Words alone can never wholly capture Truth, being always filtered by the mind which interprets them; but they can be used as a tool to guide us within. The infinite, absolute Reality can be experienced directly, thus resulting in new levels of insight and an empowered life.